VGM Opportunities Series

OPPORTUNITIES IN
MENTAL HEALTH CAREERS

Philip A. Perry

Foreword by
George Blake
President
American Association of Psychiatric Technicians, Inc.

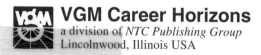

VGM Career Horizons
a division of *NTC Publishing Group*
Lincolnwood, Illinois USA

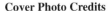

Cover Photo Credits
Clockwise from upper left: Ball State University Office of Public Information;
Lambs Farm, Libertyville, Illinois (photo by Steve Spicer); Chicago Department
of Health; Northern Essex Community College.

Library of Congress Cataloging-in-Publication Data
Perry, Philip A.
    Opportunities in mental health careers / Philip A. Perry, foreword
by George Blake.
        p.   cm. — (VGM opportunities series)
    Includes bibliographical references (p.   ).
    ISBN 0-8442-4429-5 (hbk.) — ISBN 0-8442-4430-9 (pbk.)
    1. Mental health services—Vocational guidance.   2. Mental health
services—Vocational guidance—United States.   I. Title.
. II. Series.
    RA790.75.P47   1996
    616.89'023—dc20   95-30109
                                                          CIP

Published by VGM Career Horizons, a division of NTC Publishing Group
4255 West Touhy Avenue
Lincolnwood (Chicago), Illinois 60646-1975, U.S.A.
© 1996 by NTC Publishing Group. All rights reserved.
No part of this book may be reproduced, stored in a retrieval
system, or transmitted in any form or by any means,
electronic, mechanical, photocopying, recording or otherwise,
without the prior permission of NTC Publishing Group.
Manufactured in the United States of America.

5 6 7 8 9 VP 9 8 7 6 5 4 3 2 1

CONTENTS

ABOUT THE AUTHOR

The author is a journalist who has written on health care, business, and management subjects since 1989. He was senior editor of *Health Care Strategic Management,* a national health care newsletter for two years, reporting and writing on hospital management trends, health reform, management information systems, generic pharmaceuticals, and other topics. Among his current assignments is writing medical purchasing news for American Hospital Publishing Inc., Chicago. He revised VGM's *Opportunities in Banking Careers.* His B.A. is from Northwestern University and his M.S.J. is from Medill School of Journalism.

ACKNOWLEDGMENTS

In the preparation of this book, I owe thanks to many people. Though I can't possibly mention them all, I would especially like to thank those who agreed to be interviewed. I hope the question and answer interviews in this book will provide a glimpse into the clinical and administrative work that goes on in the field of mental health care. As an outsider, even though one with a half dozen years' experience as a writer/editor in the health care field, I could not hope to convey the reality of daily life in these careers as well as the professionals themselves can and do in their own words. My contacts with them have increased my respect for their caring and helping work with the mentally ill and developmentally disabled.

I would like to thank Virginia Simon-Ashenhurst, ACSW, who made some valuable suggestions about the book. Mary Di Giovanni, president of the Council of Human Services Education, provided much useful information. So did George Blake of the American Association of Psychiatric Technicians. The editorial staff at VGM has also been an ongoing source of assistance.

Despite their efforts, there are bound to be errors remaining in the book, for which I have to take full responsibility. I hope readers will supply information to help improve any future editions.

FOREWORD

Mental health is a field in which there are many entry-level opportunities. Mental health is almost unregulated at levels below that of psychologist. Only thirty-six states license counselors, and only four states (California, Kansas, Colorado, and Arkansas) license psychiatric technicians. In the forty-six states that do not license psychiatric technicians or mental health workers, voluntary certification is available through national professional associations. In a few states, there are local associations for mental health workers.

The education needed to get into the field varies. Some facilities will hire mental health workers with no education and no experience; others require a bachelor's degree and several years' experience. But once in the field, your experience is transferable. If you have been working in a drug clinic, for instance, it is usually relatively easy to get a job working in a hospital's chronically mentally ill unit.

The one thing that you must bring to this field that cannot be taught is empathy for the fellow human beings who come under your care. Your facility or hospital may label these people as clients, patients, CMI's (chronically mentally ill), or just as a diagnosis. If you are careful not to label the people who come under your care, but rather continue to think of them as fellow human beings, and if you are careful not to take their behavior personally, then you will find this field challenging and very rewarding.

George Blake
President
American Association of Psychiatric Technicians, Inc.

CHAPTER 1

MENTAL HEALTH AND THE HELPING PROFESSIONS

The mental health professions embrace a wide variety of helping roles. From the beginning psychiatric assistant in a hospital to the top clinical and research experts in the field, people are finding rewarding careers in mental health. Karl A. Menninger, one of the pioneers of American psychiatry, said mental health is "the adjustment of human beings to the world and to each other with a maximum of effectiveness and happiness." And, in keeping with Menninger's vision, the field of mental health includes many professionals whose purpose is not only to treat illness but to restore health and then maintain it.

The mental health field is becoming increasingly specialized and it is moving at a fast pace. Millions of patients and clients need treatment, supportive services, and counseling each year. (For example, psychosis was fifth in a list of twenty-five of the most common diagnoses made by doctors, according to the March 15, 1993 issue of *Medical Benefits*.) The costs of mental illness to our society are high in both human and economic terms. However, recovery from mental illness is possible in many cases, and treatment is becoming more effective.

Many administrative and clinical specialties are part of the changing American health care scene, such as managed mental health care, human services, social work, employee assistance programs, and others. And special populations will require mental health services: the emotionally disturbed child, the pregnant teen, the mentally ill substance abuser, the homeless, the HIV infected, and so on. Many entry-level jobs exist for those with a high school education or associate degree, including:

- mental health assistant
- mental health technician
- community skills instructor
- recreational worker
- crisis prevention/intervention worker
- shelter worker
- direct service advocate
- certified nurse assistant (CNA)
- home health aide
- home health support worker
- community services worker
- child care worker
- residential counselor

These jobs are a representative sample of what beginning professionals can do in the mental health care field. Titles vary from one region of the country to another. Later chapters will discuss the general requirements for some of the many careers available.

If you're a high school student looking for a career, you can start with a list like this and discuss it with your counselor. Ask about how to become licensed or certified in your state, or wherever you want to work, in the career you choose. Mental health technicians and counselors are in demand in hospitals, community-based programs, and mental health centers nationwide. In some states they must be certified. Other states have no such requirements.

On a more advanced level, be sure you follow the program that will let you do the work you want. Do you want to do psychotherapy? Do you want to do community social work? Do you want to be in private practice? A master's degree in social work may lead to a license that allows you to bill clients for services, but a master's degree in psychology may not have third-party billing. You need to consult with knowledgeable people first, before you decide on your course of action.

Other books in the VGM Career Horizons series are devoted to the clinical specialties of psychiatrist, psychologist, and to the counseling and development fields. If you're interested in a lifetime career in the mental health field and want to know more about the training and education required for advancement, consult these books, too.

WORKING IN MENTAL HEALTH

Let's start by asking some basic questions. What would it be like to have a job in mental health? How would you start? Typical duties if you work in a hospital setting include assisting patients with activities of daily living, patient care, and feeding, as well as group recreational activities. You'll be with the patients during their day, caring for them, watching out for them, and helping them with tasks they can't do for themselves. They may spend part of the day going on a field trip or doing crafts or playing sports.

Under supervision you will be working with a team (nurses, social workers, therapists, and psychiatrists) to make sure that patients progress according to the plan for their care. If that appeals to you, you should ask yourself, What's the future after an entry-level job? What are the career paths that will lead me from just getting a job to acquiring a fulfilling vocation? Let's look at a couple of examples.

Mental health assistants are the frontline workers in psychiatric hospitals, day treatment programs, and community mental health centers around the country. Many nursing homes may have a psychiatric population of older chronic patients, too, requiring nursing assistants, aides, or CNAs. However, nursing homes are not always under the mental health system of a state, so to find these jobs requires contacts in the long-term care sector. More than 100,000 of these jobs exist in various settings. These workers may help patients in a hospital with daily activities. They are part of a psychiatric team, reporting their observations to other team members, such as nurses and psychiatrists.

Many psychiatric technicians help the developmentally disabled with basic activities of daily living—personal care, feeding, grooming—and accompany them to educational or recreational activities. In a community mental health setting, case managers may help the homeless or people in a crisis or a disaster situation. Group home managers may work in a residential setting such as a group home, where recovering people are preparing to return to normal life through "step-down" treatment under psychiatric care in the least restrictive setting possible.

A certified nurse's aide (CNA) or licensed practical nurse (LPN) may develop a psychiatric specialty. Some go on to complete a registered nurse (RN) program. They may work in a hospital or, more often than not, in an outpatient setting. A new trend is to work in a day hospital, or partial hospitalization setting, and even as a home health aide. Like mental health technicians, aides have a high level of patient contact. They carry out the treatment plans of medical specialists. The most advanced specialists may have medical training that allows them not only to assist patients with activities and observe their behavior but to do counseling or administer the psychopharmaceutical medicines that are revolutionizing treatment. Medical specialists may earn up to $30,000 or more a year.

A recreation worker might find a first job at a community center, organizing crafts or sports for people in the community. A more advanced job along this imaginary career path is that of the recreational therapist, who most likely would work for a hospital or a nursing home. He or she helps patients recover from an illness or injury by planning and engaging in an activity that's medically helpful. You might then become a therapist's assistant by getting more education and a certificate. You'd need to get an associate's degree and then pursue the certificate program of a credentialing organization like the National Council for Therapeutic Recreation. In this job category, you can expect a median income around $15,000. From there, you could go on to get a bachelor's degree and become certified as a therapist.

WHAT'S THE OUTLOOK?

If these kinds of jobs sound appealing, you probably still wonder what the future would hold, and you should take a careful look at the prospects for the field before making your decision. In the psychiatric field, there should be good prospects for employment in the future because both nursing aides and psychiatric aides are in demand and will be at least through 2005, according to government forecasts. In fact, there were more than 1,200,000 nursing aides and 100,000 psychiatric aides employed in 1992–93. What's more, many of these jobs did not even require a high school diploma. All they required was the ability to help others and to learn on the job. Of course, advancement requires more formal education and further on-the-job training.

You should familiarize yourself with the core professions of mental health—the people who run the mental health network. The team is part of a model of mental health professions that requires many different skills. The so-called core disciplines include psychologists, social workers, psychiatrists, nurses, rehabilitation and school guidance counselors, and activity therapists. As a mental health worker, you will work under the supervision of professionals who represent the core disciplines. Here's how one expert described the role of psychiatric aides in the profession:

> During the last twenty years, the contribution of paraprofessionals has gained recognition and prompted an influx of funds to college and university training programs that offer associate degrees in mental health technology and related human services fields. Graduates of these associate of arts programs (which are highly practical in nature ...) usually find positions in new career ladders established by the mental health organizations.... Because of the successful contributions of the paraprofessional in the delivery system of mental health—as well as in health corrections, and education ... mental health professionals and administrators of programs are increasingly receptive to inclusion of nonprofessionals and volunteers into its ranks of helpers.

(Sauber, Richard. *The Human Services Delivery System,* New York: Columbia University Press, 1983, p. 95.)

As a paraprofessional, you'd work with mental health practitioners who actually treat the clients or patients. Here are some brief definitions, based on the *Columbia University College of Physicians and Surgeons Complete Home Guide to Mental Health,* and the American Medical Association's *Home Medical Encyclopedia.*

Psychiatrists are physicians who treat psychological illness. They have completed medical school, a year as an intern, and three years as a resident in a medical center. As physicians, they are the only ones who can make a diagnosis and prescribe a treatment plan. This plan may consist of medication or individual or group psychotherapy. The American Psychiatric Association, Washington DC, is one of their national professional organizations.

Clinical psychologists also treat patients. They've earned a doctorate in psychology, have gone through additional training in a clinical setting with a supervisor, and then have passed licensing exams. Some choose to teach and conduct research; others become school counselors or psychotherapists. They may also become guidance counselors, marriage counselors, or rehabilitation psychologists. They conduct psychological tests, which help them assess their patients' emotional problems and determine which therapies will meet their specific needs. However, because they're nonmedical specialists, they can't prescribe drugs for treatment. The American Psychological Association, Washington, DC, is one of their larger professional associations.

Social workers help clients who are both well and ill. They sometimes specialize in mental or emotional problems. Usually, they've earned a master's degree in social work, which entails two years of graduate work plus about 900 hours of fieldwork or supervised clinical practice. They then are eligible for state licensing. They are licensed in every state, and two associations supervise professional credentialing: the National Association of Social Workers, Inc., Silver Spring, MD, and the American Board of Examiners in Clinical Social Work, Silver Spring, MD.

Psychiatric nurses specialize in psychiatry, have master's degrees, and are licensed to practice as registered nurses. They may work in a hospital or other health care facility, or they may choose to set up a private practice for psychotherapy. The American Nurses' Association, Washington, DC, certifies psychiatric clinical nurse specialists. They have to pass a qualifying exam after two years of postgraduate work and 100 hours of supervision. There are 33,000 psychiatric nurse clinicians at work nationwide.

Mental health counselors encompass a wide range of care providers. The National Academy of Certified Clinical Mental Health Counselors certifies its graduates through the American Mental Health Counselors Association, Alexandria, VA. They pass 3,000 hours of supervised practice. They can assist clients with counseling or psychotherapy.

For more information on these and other mental health topics, read about the relevant job profiles in Appendix A. You can also call or write to any of the appropriate professional associations listed at the end of each chapter.

What are the earnings prospects for the support staff who work for these professionals? Let's take for example the mental health technician at a hospital. Entry-level jobs are available to high school graduates and those with associate's degrees or baccalaureates. As you might expect, starting pay is modest. For mental health technicians at one major hospital, the pay starts at around $17,000, according to its employment director. The next level, that of licensed mental health technician, earns up to a $25,000 maximum. Above that is the senior licensed mental health technician. Salaries for this level are $18,000 minimum and $27,000 maximum. This salary range is due to experience, certification, and continuing education. The state of California pays up to $30,000 for experienced psychiatric technicians. Salaries will vary from place to place. If you find you like work as a mental health paraprofessional, advancement *will* depend on experience and continuing education.

For nurse's aides, starting pay was estimated at $8,100 to $22,400 for full-time employees in 1992–93. If you want to go beyond that, you might look into earning an LPN or RN degree in nursing. Licensed practical nursing means a commitment to a year of formal education and considerable on-the-job training from hospital staff, most likely. Still, more than 60 percent of nurses got their starting jobs not by going to a four-year college, but through an associate degree in nursing (A.D.N.). To progress and to reach the peak of the nursing profession, you'd aspire to be a registered nurse or a nurse-practitioner, with psychiatric care as your clinical specialty, which means additional training and certification. As a registered nurse, your earning power would jump dramatically—to as much as $20 an hour. Nurses are in demand throughout the country as there has been a real shortage in many regions.

OVERVIEW OF THE FIELD

Jobs in mental health can be broadly divided between the clinical and the nonclinical. Clinical workers help patients directly. Nonclinical workers deal with support services to patients. Not all mental health workers are in hospitals. Far from it. Ever since the 1970s, the trend has been away from inpatient settings for psychiatric care. That accelerated in the 1980s and 1990s with growing concern over health care costs. This will be a concern of workers for a long time to come. High turnover in the field stems in part from constant changes in mental health program funding. If social services are your goal, you've chosen one of the fastest growing fields in the country. Social services breaks down into four parts, as the government's labor department defines it: individual and family services, residential care, job training, and miscellaneous social services. Overall, the social services occupations will grow 64 percent during 1990–2005. If you're prepared for the professional and emotional demands of this important field, you may find a rewarding career in it.

Direct and Indirect Cost of Mental Illness

- U.S. economic costs of mental illness: $103.7 billion.
- Direct treatment and support costs: $42.5 billion.
- As a percentage of total personal health care spending for all illnesses: 11.5.
- Morbidity costs:[*] $47.4 billion.
- Mortality costs:[*] $9.3 billion.
- Cost of caregiver services: $4.5 billion.

---

[*]Morbidity costs: the value of lost productivity due to mental illness. Mortality costs: the lost value of productivity from premature death as a result of mental illness.

Source: Cited in *Medical Benefits* newsletter, vol. 10, no. 5, March 15, 1993.

Forecasts for Employment in Mental Health Occupations

(job totals in thousands)

Job category and number	1992	2005 projected number low to high	1992–2005 percent change low to high
psychiatric technicians	72	86 to 91	+20 to 27%
psychiatric aides	81	98 to 105	+21 to 30%
home health aides	394	794 to 835	+129 to 141%
recreational therapists	30	42	+34 to +42%
occupational therapy assistants and aides	12	21	+71 to 80%

Source: The American Work Force: 1992–2005. U.S. Dept. of Labor Bureau of Labor Statistics, April 1994. Numbers in thousands.

Fastest Growing Mental Health-Related Occupations in 1992–2005.

	Employment		Numeric	Percent
Occupation	1992	2005	change	change
Human services workers	189	445	256	136
Child care workers	684	1,135	450	66
Licensed practical nurses	659	920	261	40
Psychologists	143	212	69	48

Source: The American Work Force: 1992–2005. U.S. Department of Labor, Bureau of Labor Statistics, p. 61–64.

Where to Work

Community mental health center
Drug addiction and rehabilitation center
Residential treatment center for emotionally disturbed children
Federally funded community health center
Day hospital
General hospital outpatient psychiatric services
VA hospital
General hospital with psychiatric inpatient and/or outpatient services
Other multiservice facilities
State mental hospital
Medical school
Government health or mental health administration agency
Private mental hospital
Institute or school for mentally retarded and/or emotionally disturbed
Correctional institution or prison
Health or mental health association or foundation
College university, elementary or secondary school or school system
Alcoholism center
Nursing home

FOR MORE INFORMATION

American Board of Examiners in
   Clinical Social Work
8484 Georgia Avenue, Suite 700
Silver Spring, MD 20910

American Hospital Association
   Division of Nursing
1 North Franklin
Chicago, IL 60611

For information about nursing aides and psychiatric aides, contact:

American Mental Health Counselors
   Association
c/o American Counseling
   Association
5999 Stevenson Avenue
Alexandria, VA 22304

American Nurses' Association
600 Maryland Avenue SW
Washington, DC 20024-2571

American Psychiatric Association
1400 K Street NW
Washington, DC 20005

American Psychological Association
750 First Street NE
Washington, DC 20002-4242

Council for Standards in Human
   Service Education
Northern Essex Community
   College
Elliot Way
Haverhill, MA 01830

National Organization for Human
   Service Education
Brookdale Community College
765 Newman Springs Road
Lincroft, NJ 07738

National Association of Psychiatric
   Health Systems
National Association of Private
   Psychiatric Hospitals
Suite 1000
1319 F Street NW
Washington, DC 20004
Publishes a psychiatric hospital
   directory.

National Association of Social
   Workers, Inc.
750 First Street NE
Suite 700
Silver Spring, MD 20910

U.S. Department of Health and
Human Services Institute of Mental
Health *Mental Health Directory* lists
treatment centers nationwide. Available at government bookstores or order from:

Superintendent of Documents
   Government Printing Office
   Washington, DC 20402

CHAPTER 2

COMMUNITY MENTAL HEALTH AND HUMAN SERVICES WORKERS

Community mental health care is a model for effective and preventive care that has been adopted by the medical profession and, in many ways, by federal and state laws. It embodies the notion that a wide range of services—from preventive care to crisis intervention—should be available in the community for all those who need resources for better mental health. Community mental health care has replaced the old system of institutionalized care. It builds on the progress made in the mental health care field that allows many more patients to be deinstitutionalized and lead more normal lives. Together with new ideas about managed health care, the community model is changing the way mental health care is delivered. In short, the idea of community mental health care is to provide a whole range of services, from basic counseling to round-the-clock observation and treatment for seriously ill patients.

For the job seeker in mental health, this system of care means there are going to be fewer hospital jobs available. However, there may be more jobs in other settings. You probably won't spend your whole career working for one institution. Today, you may find more opportunities at the hospital's outpatient clinic. Or, you may find a place to start as a human services worker, a substance abuse counselor, or a recreation worker in a community agency with mental health services.

Outpatient care is for patients or clients who are capable of living on their own but need continuing attention from mental health professionals. Partial hospitalization, or day hospital treatment, is an option for some patients and is a way of saving money. Thanks to psychoactive drugs, more patients can live normal lives despite mental illnesses that once meant a life of institutionalization. However, these patients still need regular attention both to monitor their medication and to allow for counseling.

Emergency care is another vital service in any community. When a mental health crisis occurs, who can people turn to? There needs to be a resource for rapid response. Intervention centers are sometimes staffed by paraprofessionals (or beginning professionals, as they are sometimes called) and volunteers. Experience has shown their value as support staff when supervised by psychologists or psychiatrists. Crisis hotlines have saved lives.

COMMUNITY NETWORKS

It's important for mental health agencies to form a network for consultation and education. They also need to be able to make referrals. Communication between public and private agencies is vital so that no patients are neglected.

Most large American communities try to provide a wide spectrum of mental health services. Here are some of the essential services of a community mental health network (based on provisions of the Community Mental Health Centers Act of 1963):

1. Inpatient care for intensive care or treatment around the clock.
2. Outpatient care for less serious cases: adults, children, and families.
3. Partial hospitalization: at least day-care treatment for patients who can return home evenings and weekends, night care for patients able to work but needing support or lacking home arrangements.
4. Emergency care available day or night.
5. Consultation and education for other community agencies and professional personnel.

These are classified as the essential services. Other services include:

6. Diagnostic service, including both social and vocational rehabilitation.
7. Precare and after-care, with patient screening before hospitalization and home-visiting or halfway houses after hospitalization.
8. Training for all types of mental health personnel.

9. Research and evaluation of programs and addressing the problems of mental illness and treatment.

(See Richard Sauber, *The Human Services Delivery System,* pp. 101–102.)

According to current theories of mental health, most care should be given within the community. The community mental health concept has become the accepted model of care. It has been promoted through the writings of psychologists and through legislation to make it possible to develop community mental health centers. Ideally, both public and private agencies will combine to form a care network that will provide a whole spectrum of services. Of course, care begins with the most basic unit of the community, the family.

If there's a problem for a parent or a child, the whole family is affected and all family members may need counseling. It may be that a child is developmentally disabled. It's important for mental health workers to know about these disabilities. Most such workers help clients who have disabilities, not behavioral problems. In other cases, a severe behavioral problem such as chronic schizophrenia may require institutionalization. Constant care, with either medication or therapy or both, may be needed from mental health workers for such people.

THE SOCIAL SAFETY NET

In other cases, people need help with human relationships, stress, or anxiety disorders. Children may need help with education, rehabilitation, or therapy. Family members often can help each other out. Sometimes, however, they can't work out all of their problems by themselves. Perhaps there's someone close by whom they can turn to—a friend or a trusted clergyperson. But the most serious problems need the skill and perspective of a counseling professional, a family counselor, or a psychiatrist. There are many counselors with their own private practices, like doctors.

America has a longstanding commitment to public health services, and many public and community agencies staffed with social workers and crisis intervention workers were set up to help the mentally ill. It's not perfect, but it helps. From time to time, we read in the newspapers of a family tragedy, like the nineteen children in Chicago who were found alone in a filthy apartment, their parents absent, unable to care for themselves properly during the day. How are the community mental health workers to help people in these crises situations? The social safety net of public agencies operates at the local, state, and federal levels. These agencies are charged with the task of seeing that the most basic needs of families are met. This part of the government's work has a large mental health component, and human services workers are part of it.

DR. CARL BELL, CHIEF EXECUTIVE DIRECTOR

Supplementing the efforts of government agencies are community mental health groups such as the Community Mental Health Council in Chicago. This private sector agency operates under contract with state and city to provide certain services. It also contracts with HMOs and employee assistance plans. Dr. Carl Bell is its chief executive director. He discusses his interests in the field and the changing concept of community mental health today.

Q. How did you become interested in mental health?

A. I was very strong in math and science in high school, loved biology, and then when I was in college, I still took the math and biology track—and chemistry. And since I liked animal behavior and I like biology, I went to medical school. I did a rotation in psychiatry . . . and didn't like it at first, but I decided to go into psychiatry because of all the fields of medicine that I had studied, that was the one field which I had not mastered, or could not see mastering. I had not mastered surgery either, but it was real clear to me that in five years there would be no challenge there, there wouldn't be any stimulation, and to my joy, to a great extent, psychiatry has remained very much bottomless. You never fully grasp it, there's always something there to challenge you and pique your interest.

Q. You turned to community mental health. Why?

A. To people at that time, in the late sixties, in the medical school community, public health was the thing, because Kennedy had just signed the Mental Health Centers Act. The other thing is that I went to

Meharry, which is a black medical school, and that was very much in tune and in touch with public health—and community health. So it just logically followed that with the professional socialization that I had in medical school around community health and public health, as well as an interest in behavior, that community mental health would be what I would do. The thing about community health, if you're talking about careers for young people, is that first of all it includes a public health approach to mental illness, so that you're told, "Here is a community, you are responsible for this community's well-being."

Q. Does that mean a preventive approach?

A. Prevention, yes, is a big piece.

So if, for example, you're working in a black community, which I do, and you know that there's a lot of violence in that community, which in this particular black community there is, you know that there are going to be a lot of children who are at risk for developing a stress disorder, which is going to impact on their ability to learn, on their ability to have decent relationships, on their ability to refuse drugs, all of that. And if you want to be a community psychiatrist, if you're concerned with a group's health, with community health, with public health, then you look at that pattern that's going on in your community and you seek ways to ameliorate the traumatic stress that the children are under.

When community psychiatry got started, everybody was sort of hoping that they cold prevent schizophrenia, but that's stupid. We're not there yet. If we find a real hard biochemical cause for schizophrenia, it will be preventable the same way they were able to prevent phenylketonuria, the amino acid disorder. But we're not there right now.

What is preventable, in a community mental health context, are stress disorders. So when the Mississippi floods occurred—and everybody was getting stressed out—it was a perfect opportunity for someone with a community public health and mental health focus to use their skills.

Q. If a young person wants to pursue a career, yet has limited financial means, are there opportunities in mental health?

A. Things are changing so much. Now there are still roles for paraprofessionals in community mental health centers. They involve managing patients who are chronically mentally ill and need a lot of supportive therapy. So the role for paraprofessionals is around providing services for the chronic mentally ill—day activities, residential care, things like that. When you start moving into emergency mental health care, when you start moving into psychotherapy, then you're talking about needing more training.

... There's a woman I know who has a bachelor's degree, and she's just good with people. She cares about them and she's really organized, and she's mature and direct, even though she's young. She's a mental health worker where I am, and she is helping me take care of maybe sixty or seventy cases. My thing with her is, either go get a master's degree in social work, go get a Ph.D. in psychology, or go to medical school. Because, maybe it's OK to be a cog in a wheel, but I'd rather be a hub. How are you going to teach your patients to aim high if you're satisfied with being a cog? So we also encourage people to go back to school.

Q. Tell me something about the staffing that would be typical in a group like yours?

A. We've got about 140 people, maybe a third of those are administrative types who take care of buildings, personnel, people who do payroll.

We've got a couple of people with twenty years on the job in a mental health technician role, so based on their experience we gave them the equivalent of a B.A. mental health worker. Bachelor's-level folks are mental health level. Then we have master's degree workers. A master's degree in social work has a lot more clout than a master's in psychology. A master's in psychology is not a terminal degree. You cannot get licensed by the state of Illinois with a master's in psychology; you have to have a Ph.D. A master's in psychology or master's in guidance counseling does not get you officially licensed.

It depends on where you look in the organization. If you look in the outpatient and children's area, you'll see master's-level social workers, five or six of them. If you look in the adult outpatient program, where a lot of the chronic schizophrenics who are on medication come, you might see four people with bachelor's degrees, and two people with master's in social work, and the M.S.W.s get the people who have the anxiety disorders and who need some psychotherapy, while the four people who have bachelor's degrees are helping the doctor take care of long-term schizophrenics who are on medication.

If you go to the residential area, you'll see mostly bachelor's-level people; you might see somebody with a master's who's supervising seven or eight bachelor's-level folk, who are taking care of the residential facility.

If you go to the day treatment program, you might see two or three master's level supervising B.A.-level folk. Then we've got two psychologists, Ph.D.s, one doing research, one doing clinical training.

Q. What's your catchment area?

A. The south side, Avalon Park, Chatham, and the South Shore. It's a catchment area of 200,000. We're sort of a throwback to the mental health center of the sixties. What happened when the mental health center movement got dismantled and Carter lost the election was the next president, Reagan, said "OK, we're dismantling this. States, here's the money, give it out however you want to." So this whole notion of catchment aid and mental health money sort of fell down the tubes. What happened was people were still getting money but there was no coordination of services. And that's when somebody came up with the bright idea of case management.

And that's where you have someone who's a gatekeeper, and if you have a patient who needs twelve different services, residential, vocational, physical, health care, what have you, management would send them to all the separate uncoordinated services. But where I am, we've got residential, vocational, day treatment, emergency, inpatient, outpatient—we can treat the patient as one-stop shopping [as in the sixties mental health centers]. We can treat the patient for all these things. We might have to send them to different people within the organization, but they're still within the organization. That makes their life a little easier for them. So it [the community health model] has held up. We still have some need for case management. There are some people who go in and out of the hospital like crazy. Those people who go into the hospital once or twice and get it together, they can go to a clinic, they can be in vocational, they can be in a residential center, and they stay out of the hospital. But for those people who go in and out of the hospital like a rubber ball, who are using drugs, who don't have a place to live, ... they need this active case management, this assertive community treatment. And essentially, that's very intensive outpatient treatment, so they've got things happening for them to keep them out of the hospital.

Q. Where does the money come from for this?

A. The state of Illinois. They're trying to do "assertive community treatment."

Q. Describe what it's like having been in community mental health?

A. Being in community mental health, I've done organizational consulting, I'm an administrator, because I'm the CEO of the Community Mental Health Council. I know about budgets, I know about forensic psychiatry, administrative psychiatry, consultation, liaison psychiatry, inpatient psychiatry, emergency room psychiatry, geriatrics, children, alcohol, drugs, rehabilitation, victims . . . It allows me everything—private practice, psychoanalytics. I have to be a jack of all trades and nearly a master. That's a very big advantage of community psychiatry. I'll sit down with a pharmacologist and I'm up on what medication is doing to people. I can sit down with forensic psychiatrists and have intelligent discussions with them, with analysts, with child psychiatrists, geriatric psychiatrists, addictionologists.

But I'm a community psychiatrist whose job is to treat anybody who walks into his agency. I've got to have skills, and because I'm treating whoever comes in, I develop that experience, and I'm treating a high volume of patients. I've got a lot of clinical experience in many different realms. The other piece I've got in my business is academic psychiatry. I train medical students from the University of Illinois, University of Chicago, Chicago Medical School, and Osteopathic. I'm a professor of psychiatry and health at the University of Illinois.

Q. Is there any aspect of health reform that will affect mental health? Will the managed care model work well?

A. In Illinois it's too early to tell, and nationally it's difficult to tell. The problem with managed care is that they don't do very well with chronic mentally ill.

Q. For example, if an employee had an alcohol problem, would an employee assistance plan provide for alcoholism treatment?

A. For that it's pretty good, but if you're talking about high utilization of inpatient days, it doesn't quite work out. So it's really going to take another five or ten years before things get settled down. The state grant's running out.

Q. Where does that leave a community health center? Do you have to find private benefactors?

A. If you don't have that degree of sophistication to have cost accounting, and know how much it's going to cost to deliver this service, and to know that if they get into a contract that's capped, and if they say here's $1,000, take care of this chronic schizophrenic for $1,000 a year, if you've done cost accounting and you know that it costs $2,000 a year, you know if you take the contract you're going to be out of business. So the mental health centers are going to have to get very sophisticated in terms of that aspect of the business.

COUNSELING

Beyond the basics, there are many problems that may call for help from someone outside the family. Marital relationships may develop conflicts. A counselor can help a husband and wife resolve their problems, or in the case of irreconcilable differences, determine whether separation or divorce is a better solution.

Counselors in private practice deal with these problems. To become a counselor requires years of education and hundreds of hours of supervised counseling (performed under the supervision of another counselor) before they are credentialed to practice on their own. They establish their practice and become known to people in the community.

The National Institute of Mental Health (NIMH) highlighted areas of developing interest in counseling, and singled out clinical mental health counseling as a fast-growing field. Counselors head agencies that specialize in family counseling, community agency counseling, or rehabilitation counseling—all areas of growing interest, according to the surveys done for the yearbook, *U.S. Mental Health, 1994*. The American Mental Health Association, a division of the American Counseling Association, counts 12,000 counselors in its membership. Most of these are master's-level graduates of three-year clinical counseling programs. Interestingly, academic programs for counselors are attracting more women than men—about 3,300 women graduates versus 1,675 men in 1990. About 41,000 counselors are in practice now at community agencies. These agencies may also hire assistants with less than M.S.-level credentials, depending on their funding and programs. Psychosocial rehabilitation is also a growing specialty. This counseling field aims to help people return to normal life or live with their condition more effectively. Counselors develop programs that cover many therapies:

- community living skills
- recreation or socialization
- vocational rehabilitation
- case management
- education

The International Association of Psychosocial Rehabilitation Services counts 2,000 to 3,000 mostly publicly funded agencies with this specialty, dedicated to serving the seriously mentally ill. The work force is estimated to be 32,000 counselors. Since each agency has a staff of sixteen on average, the opportunities are there for case workers as well as mental health workers with a human services interest. Indeed, the growth of partial care and multiservice mental health organizations has been very strong over the last twenty years, with more than 28,000 mental health workers with less than B.A.-level education as of 1990. (See table, Where the Jobs Are, at the end of this chapter.)

FUTURE TRENDS

A future trend in community health is outpatient care for people with mental disorders. Where possible, patients will be cared for in their homes and in the "therapeutic community." This is increasingly possible with the use of medications and therapy. It's a new frontier, and it may represent the biggest future growth area for mental health. Certainly, if geriatric care is included, the home and the community will be the major health care setting in many programs.

This chapter has concentrated on the mental health support network in this country and the people who run it—psychiatrists, social workers, and counselors. In the next few chapters, the opportunities for B.A. and less-than-B.A. jobs will be treated in detail.

Entry-level jobs:

- paraprofessional with a counselor in agency or private practice
- entry-level social workers

Upper-level jobs:

- clergy
- counselor
- social worker

Top-level jobs:

- psychologist
- psychiatrist

Where the Jobs Are

Number of Mental Health Workers with Less Than a B.A. Degree in Various Job Settings.

	1972	*1976*	*1978*	*1986*	*1988*	*1990*
In all mental health organizations	140,379	n/a	139,101	114,149	132,786	142,345
In state and county mental health hospitals	99,791	94,531	86,056	64,220	67,343	64,163
In private psychiatric hospitals	5,594	7,317	7,309	8,234	12,693	11,531
In psychiatric services of nonfederal general hospitals	10,270	12,738	12,565	10,915	13,576	15,195
In VA medical centers	12,208	12,097	12,328	5,777	7,013	7,461
In residential treatment centers for emotionally disturbed children	4,561	4,834	5,640	7,547	10,451	14,937
In freestanding outpatient psychiatric clinics	1,136	2,170	2,440	301	906	572
In freestanding partial-care and multiservice mental health organizations	816	879	1,158	17,155	20,804	28,486

Source: U.S. Mental Health, 1994, table 6.8a–g.

FOR MORE INFORMATION

American Association for Marriage and Family Therapy
    1717 K Street NW
    Washington, DC 20006

American Association of Pastoral Counselors
    9508A Lee Highway
    Fairfax, VA 22031

National Association for Counseling and Development
    5999 Stevenson Avenue
    Alexandria, VA 22304

(Subdivisions include the American Counseling Association, the American School Counselor Association, and the American Mental Health Counselors Association.)

Visiting Nurse Associations of America
    Association of Psychiatric Nurses
    National Nurses Society on Addictions
    3801 E. Florida, Suite 900
    Denver, CO 80210

CHAPTER 3

PSYCHIATRIC TECHNICIAN

To visualize yourself as a mental health worker, picture yourself in the following situations, which include the highs and lows of the job. First, suppose you're a mental health technician in a hospital. You've worked with an inpatient, Joe, for two weeks after he was admitted to the hospital for depression. You've accompanied him to group therapy sessions, worked with him in activities, perhaps even observed him in isolation if he was considered suicidal. Now he's beginning to recover, thanks to therapy and medication. He'll be released and his treatment will "step down" gradually to day hospital and home care, and if he recovers fully, he'll return to normal life.

Or, imagine you're a home health aide. You're visiting Jane, an elderly patient who is one of four or five patients you'll see today. You help her with routine activities of the day while following a treatment plan developed by a team of specialists, including a psychiatrist, from your agency. They recommended that you accompany your patient on a shopping trip to help her overcome her fear of leaving home. After a successful outing, she thanks you for your help. Her family is grateful, too, knowing that you're trained to care for the physical and psychological problems related to aging.

Suppose you're working in a community mental health center. You take a call on the crisis line and support a teen who's taken more drugs than he can handle. Later he visits your drop-in program and begins to get active in after-school youth activities like midnight basketball. You can see the improvement as he straightens out his life and develops new interests.

Now comes the downside. For a mental health worker, the lows may come when a hospital patient doesn't respond to therapy, or when an unruly patient disrupts the whole unit, requiring restraint and isolation.

A home health aide may find a patient's home in a mess, or be confronted with a confused patient who is angry at her loss of independence and takes the anger out on the aide. With the two of you alone in a home, there's no one to solve the problem for you. Or an alcoholic patient may have to be treated for sprains from a fall or cigarette burns when he fell asleep smoking. You may not get thanks for your help; in fact, you may find the patient resents you.

A substance abuse worker may hit a low point when one of her recovering clients drops out of the recovery program and returns to drug use. She may blame herself for failure to reach that individual and pull her out of her downward spiral.

These situations are fictional, but they're based on the reality of the field—high emotional involvement and possible burnout. Employers are looking for people who enjoy the helping aspects of the work and can handle the daily stress levels that go with the mental health professions.

TERESA BELLO-JONES, JD, RN

One way to prepare for a career in this kind of field is to take an associate degree program that is available in many states and required in some. As an example, look at the California state requirements for psychiatric technician, a job that attracts many kinds of people like single parents, ex-servicemen and women from the military corps, and career-changing workers who are attracted to health care. These jobs can pay up to $30,000 or more a year in California.

How do the psychiatric technicians for this statewide system of mental health care gain their credentials? Teresa Bello-Jones, JD, RN, is executive officer of the Board of Vocational Nurse and Psychiatric Technician Examiners, Sacramento, CA. She supplied information used here, which draws on the board's publication, *Licensed Psychiatric Technician, An Occupational Guide,* and its fact sheets on psychiatric technicians and vocational nurses. Training requirements were current as of December 1994.

Q. What are the job prospects in mental health for the next ten years?

A. Job opportunities for psychiatric technicians will continue in state hospitals/centers of the mentally disordered and developmentally disabled, residential care facilities for the developmentally disabled, sheltered workshops, psychiatric hospitals, correctional institutions, day treatment centers, and clinics for alcoholic and chemically dependent clients.

Q. What education will be required of mental health workers? of psychiatric technicians? of nurses?

A. Psychiatric tech programs in California require 1,530 hours of training, or a full-time program length of twelve to fourteen months; part-time programs require eighteen to twenty-four months. Course content ranges from psychology and pharmacology to developmental disabilities, nursing, and other areas of study. Most psych tech programs are in community colleges (nine programs, 64 percent of students); hospital-based programs (three programs, 22 percent of students); and two adult programs (14 percent of students).

Licensed vocational nurses require 1,530 hours of a training curriculum with a wide ranging course load from anatomy and psychology to nursing processes, leadership, and supervision. Vocational programs are found in community colleges (forty-three programs with 58 percent of all students); fifteen adult programs with 20 percent of students; nine private schools serving 12 percent of students; and other programs for a total of seventy-four programs in all. Also there are twenty more vocational nurse programs awaiting accreditation.

Q. What job skills are most in demand?

A. Professional expectations for psychiatric technicians in hospitals: "They are concerned with all details of the client's daily life and their effect on physical, mental, and emotional well being."

Technicians assist with eating, sleeping, recreation, rehabilitation. Techs are concerned with clients' development of work skills. Many techs work in community mental health agencies, which provide day treatment, crisis intervention, drug and alcohol detoxification, and counseling. They assist in all the agency services mentioned:

- make home visits to people who are clients
- have sound judgment with clients

- know when to refer the client for more specialized care or professional assistance
- have good communication skills
- know about social interactions
- use these skills to help clients who are living outside the hospital setting
- give basic nursing care to clients (take and record temperature, pulse, respiration, blood pressure; give medication; provide physical care)
- observe clients' behavior carefully
- counsel and train clients for daily living
- work closely with psychiatrists, psychologists, psychiatric nurses, and psychiatric social workers

You may be interested to know that the typical salary range of a psychiatric technician is $15 to $17 per hour, or $28,800 to $32,640 a year in California, according to information from the state's certifying agency, the Board of Examiners. A licensed vocational nurse, or LVN, may earn $13 to $16 per hour or $24,960 to $30,720 per year.

Although hospitals are one of the most common places for psychiatric personnel to work, they're not the only job settings. In California, they're also at work in developmental centers, day treatment centers, correctional facilities, and psychiatric technician educational programs, as well as in state hospitals and psychiatric hospitals and clinics.

Each state has its own licensing requirements for health care facilities. California, as one of four states that required licensure of psychiatric technicians, has a higher than average education requirement. *Other states may begin to require licenses as part of a national trend to more educational requirements and certification in the health professions. This has already happened in the counseling profession.*

Your education plans—as a mental health worker, nurse, therapy assistant, or other vocation—should be geared to meet the requirements for the locale where you plan to work. Some states have reciprocal agreements with surrounding states, meaning that they've coordinated their licensing so that health care professionals can move to other states and their licensure will be recognized immediately, or after approval.

MENNINGER CLINIC

What would it take to get a job in one of the country's top private psychiatric care facilities? Menninger is considered to be such a center of excellence. In an interview with Tim McManus, director of employee relations at Menninger Clinic, it becomes clear that training is important for advancement in the mental health field.

Q. Describe the nature of the work that a mental health worker does at Menninger?

A. For mental health workers, they escort and supervise patients to and from activities. They act as sounding boards for patients. They work with the patient in planning leisure and unstructured time. They're not doing therapy, but they're on the front line and observe patient behavior. They report the patient behavior back to their treatment team, to a social worker/psychiatrist and other team members.

Counselors take a more active role in activities of daily living. Some are treatment coordinators for patients who are living in the community. [Patients are in group settings during some days with special activities.] Activity therapists in our hospital are in degreed positions. A music therapist, horticulture therapist, and a recreation therapist—they have to have a bachelor's degree at a minimum.

Q. What are the working conditions in the hospital?

A. It's a forty-hour week. We do have some part-time. Three shifts each work forty hours a week, seven days a week.

Q. What training is needed for the mental health workers themselves at entry level?

A. Experience—for mental health workers. There *is* a career ladder at this institution. Mental health worker is an entry-level position. Educational requirements are a high school diploma or a G.E.D., and prior experience working in a mental health setting. Here in Topeka we have, for example, Topeka State Hospital, the VA hospital, and a number of mental health centers. Some college course work in psychology is preferred.

Q. Are there many with degrees coming into the hospital?

A. Some college students are working here while pursuing a degree. Some work here if they are thinking about a career in mental health to see if this is what they're cut out for. Some work here before graduate school, to see if they want to go on, before they get a master's or a Ph.D. It's a great way for them to find out.

Q. What's the range of entry-level jobs with a mental health care component in the hospital, e.g., psychiatric aides, nurses aides, LPN nursing?

A. Mental health workers, activity therapists, child care workers, some counseling jobs, licensed practical nurse. The salary for child care workers and the mental health workers would be about the same, about $14,500, $17,000 midpoint, $19,500 maximum. There are also counselors in our partial hospitalization program. More advanced jobs are counselor 1–2–3. Degrees are usually required.

The next step up is licensed mental health technician. Salaries are $17,000 minimum, $21,000 midpoint, $25,000 maximum. They have to complete an associate degree from a school [with a specialized program] like Washburn University in Topeka.

Q. What are their duties? How do they differ from entry level?

A. Primarily LMHT's can dispense medication; mental health workers can't.

The next step is senior licensed mental health technician. Salaries are $18,000 minimum, $23,000 midpoint, $27,000 maximum. The difference is experience, more than anything else; again they have to have this mental health worker program associate degree and three years' experience as a mental health worker. They train and supervise workers and technicians.

Q. Beyond that, what career options are there at Menninger?

A. There are a few partial-hospitalization services positions; there's a career ladder there, too. Counselor-level one does not require a B.A.; counselor two does; counselor three requires a master's degree.

Q. What career options are there at your outpatient centers?

A. We have halfway houses and what we call community residence programs in the community. Basically the counselors are centrally located on our main campus. The people who live and work in the halfway houses are house managers and assistant managers. Mostly they're there to prepare the meals, to be a listening ear, but the therapy is done by the counselors on the main campus for individual therapy and group therapy.

Q. What are the typical earnings?

A. For these after-care counselors, the salaries for this level are $19,500 to $27,200 for counselor one, $25,000 to $35,000 for counselor two, $31,000 to $45,000 for counselor three.

Q. What do the counselors do?

A. Counselors are needed in partial hospitalization services. Halfway houses have managers and assistant managers. One couple lives in. Others help with preparation of meals. [The patients often live in the halfway houses and] then patients are treated in a central location at the main campus for therapy. The education levels for these jobs are counselor one, no B.A.; counselor two, B.A.; counselor three, M.S.

Q. What is the job outlook?

A. The job outlook is still pretty good. At entry level, we do need a lot of people. I don't know about the rest of the country, but around here, it seems everyone is trying to do more with less. The work is done by fewer clinicians. We're a closed-staff hospital. We have a significant number of psychiatrists who work here full-time but fewer than in the past. They're functioning as leaders who still do group therapy and individual therapy. In addition to the psychiatrists, we are working with fewer psychologists and social workers.

In the past, patients were often hospitalized for six months. Now twenty-five to thirty days is [the average]. The employees have to connect with patients and do good work [in a much shorter time period]. So the psychiatrist has to monitor medication closely. They've got their hands full with this rapid turnover.

Q. Obviously, Menninger's is a top destination for people who want work, but are there other places if Menninger's has no openings?

A. Yes, Topeka State, the VA Hospital, community mental health centers. They'll go there and get some experience; then they'll come here and apply for work. I think the working conditions here are a little better than some other places.

JAY SALTER, PSYCHIATRIC TECHNICIAN

A psychiatric technician can choose many specialties. Jay Salter chose forensic work at Atascadero State Hospital in California. He also is president of the California Association of Psychiatric Technicians. He discusses his experiences and education, as well as the trends in the field today.

Q. Can you describe your background, education, and training that led you into the field of psychiatric technician?

A. I have a B.A. in English lit, I worked for a number of years right after college, I was editing a newspaper in Vietnam for Pacific Architects and Engineers, an engineering company. I came back from that job and worked with the Jet Propulsion Laboratory, and after that job ended it was a good opportunity to move away from Los Angeles, so we decided to come the central coast and build our own house on our own land. It so happened that Atascadero State Hospital was within five minutes' drive from our house. And I went there and applied for a job and subsequently became a licensed psychiatric technician by going to school right there on the campus of the hospital facility. The schooling was provided by Cuesta Community College, and they offered the psych tech course. Every year they graduated a number of students who would go to work right there at Atascadero.

Q. Did the job meet your expectations?

A. I had no idea what it would be like, but once I did get involved I found it fascinating. Here I was, a person who had an arts background, working in what seemed to me a scientific field; and we were encouraged to become very active in leading group therapy sessions, to become proficient in making client assessments and symptomology and so forth, and so I thought, wow, this is really a very fascinating thing....

Q. Would psych techs today have the same opportunity?

A. Sure. They've limited to a certain extent—the ability for psych techs to be as free-ranging as we used to be.... I think they could run these hospitals a lot more economically if they would utilize psychiatric technicians as fully as their training and qualifications would allow.

When we first did this in the mid-1970s, I had a group of eight patients for whom I was the chief sponsor on my shift, and it was my responsibility to present my patients in an interdisciplinary team setting, where I wrote up the entire review of the patient's conduct and behavior from one end to the other, and made the presentation just as though I was almost a resident or intern.

Q. How does Atascadero differ from the typical experience and training of a psych tech?

A. The great majority of California psych techs work with developmentally disabled, they work not in state hospitals, but in developmental centers. They're treating primarily the mentally retarded—profoundly disabled people who in many cases can't care for themselves at all. You have to teach them to feed themselves. You have to work with people who will never be able to feed themselves, and they have to be kept clean; you're dealing with what amounts to perpetual children. The people I know who work in that area become very involved with their care and their lives.

Q. Is that wise?

A. You have to. I don't see how you can avoid it because the psychiatric technicians are the ones who put their hands on the clients. That's what differentiates us from all the other disciplines. We're the ones who have to treat the patients day in and day out, twenty-four hours a day. Everyone else comes to work at 8:00 in the morning and goes home at 4:00 in the afternoon, but the psych techs are there all twenty-four hours. And they're the ones who put into practice the orders that the physicians give, or the psychologists or the "professional" who's overseeing the therapy; whatever those orders are, we put it into practice; we make it real.

Q. What was most rewarding about your work?

A. What was most rewarding was getting a client in there who could actually make progress, and turn around, and I can remember two or three I was involved with in my particular group who were actually able to get back onto the street in the course of about a year's time. And I know that it was a successful experience, because the clients sent letters back to our unit from time to time saying how grateful they were—for the therapy they received, for the new chance that they'd been given in their lives.

Q. What therapy helped turn them around?

A. Well, it was the fact that there were people who really cared about them as human beings, as unique individuals, and made a commitment to really push them to such an extent that they would have to recognize they'd have to make certain changes in their lives.

Q. Was this evident to them through group or individual therapy?

A. Yes. Through the group therapy, but I think mostly through the individual contact with them. Because you're not just dealing with them in the group setting, but in the dining room, the day hall, at night watching television. You are there as a parent figure more than anything else. You're modeling conduct for them.

Q. What are the current trends in the field?

A. Everything is in flux. There's a great pressure to economize. Our governor, Pete Wilson, is doing everything he can to cut the cost of government. And one of the easier ways to cut is to reduce the size of the developmental centers and the mental hospitals and figure out ways to get these people who once were treated exclusively in the institutions out onto the street. That is primarily a good idea, though a lot of people I work with wouldn't think so. Because it means the jobs aren't going to be there at the state hospitals. There's just an enormous amount of work to be done in a variety of settings, out there in the community and in the counties. I think county mental health is going to begin expanding the areas where its psychiatric technicians can work.

I've talked to a number of developmental centers which are interested in employing psychiatric technicians much the way registered nurses are employed in a home health setting, where they would travel to where patients lived in their communities and help treat them right in the home settings.

Q. Would they be able to administer medication?

A. Yes.

Q. Are there any liabilities to worry about?

A. If you're working for the state or for a county, you're probably covered for liability.

Q. What are the advantages of treating them in a less-restrictive environment?

A. There are two reasons. One is money. It's very expensive to maintain them in an institution, in a developmental center, or a mental hospital, which can run as high as $80,000 to $100,000 per client. If you can get them out onto the street and living in the community in a place that you don't have all that overhead, to a place where you can still maintain them and treat them, it's going to cost less money. Plus, a lot of people believe that by mainstreaming them, you're putting them in a place and requiring responsibilities of them that are therapeutically beneficial for them. If you put them in an institution and keep them in, to a certain extent they'll never recover.

Q. So the therapeutic community is valid?

A. Yes, though a lot of people I work with hesitate to agree.

Q. What would you recommend to people going into the field today? What is the right training, and what can they expect from a career?

A. Of course I would recommend that they have at least a high school diploma. You're not going to get very far without a high school diploma, at least here in California. That's the basic requirement. Beyond that, I would simply say that this is an excellent first rung of the ladder, in terms of getting involved with the mental health business as a career. I have a number of friends who started out as psychiatric technicians who have since become registered nurses or social workers, or rehab therapists, who've gone on to take training beyond the entry-level license. And it's a wonderful experience. This is a wonderful way of getting people off welfare and into jobs that are paying a living wage.

Q. About pay, in California's state-paying jobs the pay is good, about $15 to $17 an hour. Is that realistic? $28,000 to $32,000 a year?

A. Yes, for the state-paying jobs, that's realistic. It falls off from there. The counties pay less, and in private industry they pay less.

JANICE O'NEILL, PSYCHIATRIC TECHNICIAN

As Jay Salter pointed out, most psychiatric technicians work with the developmentally disabled. This population is treated at state hospitals such as Sonoma Developmental Center, Sonoma, CA, where Janice O'Neill is a psychiatric technician, Sonoma chapter president, and statewide vice president, California Association of Psychiatric Technicians.

Q. What is your background? How did you get interested in this profession?

A. I was a single parent looking for a way to support my family without minimum wage jobs, and decided to go back to school. And I discovered the psych tech program. At that time it was a really concentrated junior college program, twenty units a quarter. It was one year, hard-core, nonstop, Monday to Friday, 8:30 to 5:00 of concentrated effort to get through school.

Helping people is an attitude that all of us psych techs have; trying to help people seemed to satisfy that part of me. And it didn't take forever to get through school. And I learned how to work on a team of professionals, psychologists, psychiatrists, social workers, recreational therapists, occupational therapists, registered nurses, social workers. We worked as a team, once I became employed, to decide what was best for the total care of one individual with developmental disabilities, or mentally ill people. I got interested because of my own personality, wanting to help people, and my own financial need.

Q. When you got through with school, did you find there was work that you'd been trained for?

A. When I looked for work, there was plenty of work. I went to work with autistic children. I worked for the first four years with autistic children. It was quite an experience. It was very difficult, and very draining emotionally—exhausting physically and emotionally—but it was the most rewarding work I think I've ever done. That was at Napa State Hospital at the children's center. They had just gotten a grant and just started an autistic program. They first had to identify the children at the center that they could diagnose as autistic. And so it was a well-staffed, well-run program. I got in on the ground floor. And it was probably one of the largest in the nation at that time.

Q. Eventually you moved on and came to Sonoma?

A. I moved on from autistic children, to chronic schizophrenic, undifferentiated type, that's a catch-all. People who had been there, that was the end of the road for them. They had been through every treatment setting, every type of boarding-care home and mental health facility, and they finally wound up at the state hospital. They had been there for a long time and they were lifers, chronic people, mentally ill. And I worked on the coed unit or ward, and then I worked in the all-female ward. I had a lot of experience with the hard-core mentally ill. When you're working in this field you see it all. You learn how to handle yourself in any situation. This job was interesting because once you become a psych tech, you can do anything; you have to do anything. It's an education in itself.

I worked as a psych tech outside state service in Butte County Mental Health, for the county at a PHF, a psychiatric health facility, and that was one of the twelve original residential treatment centers that the state developed.

It's a nineteen-bed residential treatment center. My title was mental health nurse. And you had to be a psych tech to hold that position. I was in charge of health care aides. Many of them had four- and five-year degrees in social service or a bachelor's in business or anything else. They were working to get themselves through school. I was in charge of them.

Q. What did you think of that center compared to the big state hospital?

A. It was a world of difference. In fact when I went back to the state hospital it was a pretty difficult transition. The state imposes a three-day hold on someone who is a danger to themselves, or a danger to others, or gravely disabled and unable to care for themselves. We'd get all kinds of people, mostly people who'd been rejected—or homeless—from state hospitals or state institutions who'd wander the streets. And they'd live in boarding care homes; they'd stop taking their medication. Or college students, just before finals, they'd get suicidal,... or people who would go berserk, they'd go to the local hospital, and they'd come into Butte County psychiatric health facility for an assessment. I would assess their condition, in a psychological evaluation, and I would take medication orders from the psychiatrist. I could give medications. And that was an interesting experience and I pretty much was in charge of that. So when I went back to the institutional setting, it was more like I wasn't in charge of anything; I was in charge of my group of mentally ill or disabled people.

Q. Which situation worked better for you?

A. It didn't make any difference to me personally; I'm still the same person and I have the same license. It spanned such a great field, I can do so much with my license, that was a different occupation basically with the same title.

Q. At Sonoma, what is it like working with the developmentally disabled population?

A. The developmental center is just a whole different world. You know they're not called patients here, they're called clients or consumers in the developmental centers. And we deliver services to them. It took me a while to start calling these people with mental disabilities "clients." It's a different world in that they're completely helpless, compared to the mental health people, who are at times very lucid and very normal, until you notice that they're crazy. But the disabled people have cerebral palsy, they have physical deformities, they're in wheelchairs, they're bed patients. There's a lot of medical attention required. This is the largest facility in the state. There are so-called units or residences. You have certain residences, one of which is a nursery; we get crack babies, which is real sad, young children who are born disabled and need all kinds of medical intervention just to keep them alive physically.

And we work as a team to give our input to help to control them, and we have team meetings to review their medication all the time. The developmental center is real interesting, divided into two groups. There are the nursing facility units, SNF or skilled nursing facility, which are units where you have nursing. The clients are in wheelchairs, with chronic physical disabilities. And then you have ICF units, intermediate care facility units. And these ICF units are behavior units. And you've got this split in the center, half works with behaviors and the other half works with disabilities.

Q. What would be an example of a "behavior"?

A. Somebody who's banging their head against the wall until it bleeds or splits open or who assaults their peers or attacks the staff or beats somebody over the head with a chair. Those are pretty serious, severe behaviors.

Q. What would the team do?

A. They would get together and decide the best program to work on these behaviors. And the psych tech would have the most input because they live with this person eight hours a day, sometimes sixteen hours a day if there's overtime.

Q. What would you recommend?

A. One of my clients can move one arm from her elbow to her wrist, she can move it to the right. So after I dressed this person, which is very difficult because she's stiff as a board, I would do a range of motion exercises with her to stretch her muscles. I would uncurl her fingers and curl them and massage them. And I would take her and put her in a wheelchair and position her in a custom-molded wheelchair, and put her on a tram . . . which carries clients to the classroom, and then, attend the classroom with the person, and since she could only move the one arm, to place a switch in front of her and give her a choice, through pictures, of what activity she wanted, depending on which switch she would push, whether it was to turn on a tape player—we discovered that she liked to listen to music. And each time she would push the one switch that would give her the music she liked, and each time we would move that switch a little farther so she would have to reach and flex that almost-atrophied muscle. And at the same time keep her happy and notice when she was sad and keep her clean and groomed.

It's a very challenging job. You go from the residents' bathing, grooming, dressing, dining, to the educational-vocational part of the person, and then you record data all the way, and train them, and whatever they're able to do you help them develop. Whether it's pushing a switch, or standing and walking in a walker with assistance from point A to point B, or learning how to use the toilet. Toilet training somebody who's thirty-five years old—and they do learn how to use the toilet. They've never been trained! It's very frustrating because it's very slow, but they do learn and it's rewarding when you see someone actually learn and be able to take care of themselves.

My favorite thing is a person who was placed in an institution when she was ten and who knows why she was placed there. I finally was able to speak to her parents, and they said she had stopped talking to them and she stopped responding to them. Since I'd had my experience at Napa with autistic children and since a lot of those children I worked with were deaf, I immediately, as soon as I was introduced to this person at Sonoma, I asked how long has she been deaf? And they laughed and said, "Oh, she's not deaf. She just listens when she wants to."

And I persisted for two years demanding that she be tested. Finally they had to give her medication and I had to restrain her for twenty minutes so they could test her, and she was deaf. After talking to the parents, they discovered she had massive scarring on her eardrums, and had had a childhood illness before penicillin. And she'd ended up in a developmental center and she'd been there for over forty years. Once the staff realized she was deaf, the world opened up for her. It was too late for her because she was socially retarded by then, but she goes to class everyday and uses a mixer and a blender and does all sorts of things. And that was because of me. That is the kind of thing we can do.

Q. Obviously you need persistence. What other qualities do you need to be a psych tech?

A. I would look for someone who is mentally very stable, very realistic, and who is kind. That's important to me. If I were going to hire someone to work with these helpless people, I would look for patience and a lot of empathy. I would look for somebody who was articulate and could read and write, because documentation is important in an institution. Someone straight out of high school, it would be scary because they don't have enough experience with people. Because it is scary. You need to be able to accept people for what they are with or without their disabilities. Because you're faced with things that a normal person would run from.

Q. In what situations is there physical challenge or danger?

A. In the skilled nursing unit you don't have to worry about confrontations because they're confined to wheelchairs. However, they can assault you, and I know people who've been just flat taken out. Our workmen's comp rate is very high. It's about 6 to 8 percent of the entire developmental services work force. As opposed to California Youth Authority, which is 3 percent, now state hospitals is 8 to 10 percent, which is second only to Highway Patrol. [Author's note: By way of comparison, in 1993 the Occupational Safety and Health Administration reported health services' rate of injuries and illnesses at 9.1 cases per 100 workers. Nursing and personal care facilities had the highest illness and injury rate: 17.3 per 100 workers in 1993 and 18.6 in 1992.] So those people better stay in shape—the people in the developmental centers who work with the ICF or behaviors, or who work with patients who are . . . ambulatory. You are in danger in some of these places. These people are not only physically capable of killing you, but they're retarded, you can't reason with them, they don't understand. So you have to know what you're doing and work your programming and do what you're supposed to do with them. It's a very challenging job.

Q. Do you think the training is adequate? Are you pushing for changes?

A. Yes, we are working with the educators toward some changes to keep pace with what's going on in today's society.... We'll be working with them to develop different types of training. You get a full range, medically. You can change tracheostomies, you can do catheterization, you can do injections, basic nursing, blood pulse, vital signs, respiration. You can walk into a room and irrigate someone's catheter, and go in the next room and be involved in a five-man takedown. And you've got the same license that covers both of those things.

Q. Once you get to a facility where you'll work, is there facility-specific training?

A. Yes. That's a requirement.

Q. Is there continuing education?

A. Yes. And our union is responsible for that. We had to fight to get that in order to be recognized as a profession. And now we've only just recently established the continuing education. We need thirty units every two years, and basically anything that's accepted by the American Nursing Association or anything that's related to the job whether it's death and dying, geriatrics, treatment of drug and alcohol abuse; the range is a very broad spectrum.

Q. This is not a routine job?

A. It's certainly not routine!

Q. Do you see the future of psych techs expanding?

A. I see the psych techs field expanding. I see psych techs going into corrections. I'd like to see psych techs expanding to other states. There are three other states psych techs are licensed in; there probably will be more. There's a lot of mentally ill people out there.

Q. What are earnings like for a psych tech?

A. In January 1994, the starting salary would have been $2,204 a month at a state facility. There's a range, A, B, and C. Range B is $2,293–$2,768 (after fifteen college credits). Range C is $2,385–$2,898. As a senior psych tech at range C you can make more than that, over $3,000 a month.

Q. California is one of the biggest states; do you have a lot of mobility during a career?

A. Yes. Over half of us are not employed by the state. We just work independently, or I worked in the county. You can work for the county, or work in the community.

FOR MORE INFORMATION

Contact your state department of mental health or your state mental health association for information about accredited training programs.

American Association of Psychiatric Technicians
P. O. Box 14014
Phoenix, AZ 85063-4014

A nonprofit association representing and serving psychiatric technicians in every state. Provides certification for psychiatric technicians. Membership: 1,500.

American Psychiatric Nurses Association
1200 Nineteenth Street NW
Suite 300
Washington, DC 20036

Foundation for Hospice and Homecare
519 C Street NE
Stanton PK
Washington, DC 20002

This organization provides information and accredits homemaker-home health aides.

National Association of State Mental Health Directors
66 Canal Center Plaza
Suite 302
Alexandria, VA 22314

National Organization for Human Services Education
Box 6257
Fitchburg State College
Fitchburg, MA 01420

Psychiatric Technician, Guidance Chronicle Publications, is available from counseling offices, high schools, for sale, or call the publisher at 315–497–0330.

CHAPTER 4

HOME HEALTH AIDE

The home health aide or home health support worker is among the fastest-growing job categories in health care. Several factors are driving up demand for these workers. First, the U.S. population is aging and more and more seniors need help at home with daily living or with medication, therapy, or other health care needs. Second, the federal government has thrown its support behind the move to home care, with Medicare, Medicaid, the Older Americans Act, and Social Services Block Grants, all major government programs that fund health care. Home care is often less expensive than hospital care or skilled care in a nursing home, so it's to the advantage of health care providers and payers to find the least expensive method of care. Then, too, seniors do not like to leave the homes they've known their whole lives for the uncertainties of life in a nursing home. Seniors and their families often choose home care as a good compromise.

In caring for children, it is also possible that home health care can save money and improve the patient's outlook. It's predicted that child care work will be a growth industry through to the twenty-first century. Home health aides may find an opportunity here, too. Not all home health aides are mental health workers, but for many, mental health training becomes vital for their work with their homebound patients. According to health care professionals, this can be a good beginning to a health care career with a mental health component. But the more responsibility they take on, the more training they'll need, if quality is to be maintained.

Training requirements for home health aides are often minimal. For some aide jobs, there is not even a requirement for a high school education. However, active care of patients demands adequate training in mental health assistance. Some training is required by states, and more is recommended by professional associations. The National HomeCaring Council (now part of the Foundation for Hospice and Homecare) developed a program for home health aides for the elderly. You'll take sixty hours of classroom and laboratory instruction and fifteen hours of field practice as part of this program, which is intended to improve the quality of care. Some agencies require such training and screen their workers to make sure they are either trained already or willing to go through an approved program. The need for more workers at all skill levels is made clear in the statistics of senior care: by one estimate, seven million older persons needed help each year in the 1980s, but the entire mental health system only treated seven million clients a year of all ages in those years.

JEAN FLAWS-CHERVINKO, HOME HEALTH
AIDE COORDINATOR

One program that's been active in home care is Rush Home Care Network, Chicago, where Jean Flaws-Chervinko is a coordinator of home health aides. She sees opportunities ahead for aides with mental health training, both at the entry level for home health aides, and for more highly trained individuals such as psychiatric nurse specialists.

Q. Ms. Flaws-Chervinko, can you describe what you're doing with Rush Home Care Network in Chicago and tell me about the changes in mental health care settings toward home health care?

A. My background is I'm a nurse. Right now I coordinate the home health aide program at Rush, which is the CNAs (certified nurse's aide) working within the home. Since we're a Medicare-based agency, we provide intermittent visits underneath a clinician's care plan. Usually the clinician is a nurse, sometimes a therapist also. Since I have taken this position, we have definitely tripled the amount of home health aide usage that we have. And basically a home health aide under Medicare regulations is a CNA who goes out to a home and really provides some type of personal care for the patient, meaning assistance with ADLs (activities of daily living) and such. Previously, anybody with a psych background, like a psych nurse, felt it wasn't a very good idea to have anybody [treated] in the home because they sometimes sabotaged the plan of their care [if they weren't in a hospital setting]. We found that by having consistent home health aides and in-servicing them on some of the psych diagnoses and mental health issues, that we were able to complement the care plan quite a bit. Probably almost a third of the home health aide visits we do are with psych patients. That's worked well, in-servicing a certain group of people with all aspects (of psychiatric care). Most of the aides will say that someone doesn't have to have a mental illness diagnosis but will probably still have some components of one just because they are elderly and out in the community.

So I definitely see that it's growing in everything we see statistics-wise about CNAs: cost-effectiveness, how significant they will be in the next couple of years, and how their profession is going to increase.

Q. What's the training for a CNA?

A. A CNA receives training, either from a nursing home that provides courses or from a community college or one of the medical tech colleges. They get 120 hours of clinical training, Illinois is a little higher; it's individual with all the states. Once they receive that, they can go ahead and work as a CNA in a hospital, although hospitals don't always require them to be certified.

Q. Would it be an associate degree?

A. No it's a certificate. They're under the professional licensure, and the state recognizes them.

Q. Do CNAs sometimes come right out of high school and go into training?

A. Yes. You don't even need a high school education for this, believe it or not. In this day and age most places do want you to get an equivalent (G.E.D.) but technically, according to the regulations, they do not need a high school education. Once they receive the training they are recognized through the Illinois department of public health and they're put on the list as recognized and qualified.

Q. How do people get a specialty in psychiatric care after starting in a program like this?

A. Now they would be attracted to us mainly because we have a strong psych nurse program, and they would be able to function with patients with mental health diagnoses. We have to offer twelve hours of in-service a year. I regulate what our clients needs are or their diagnoses and give them tools the home health aides can work with, so that our in-servicing program would gear toward mental health education.

Q. What would a day's work be like when they are seeing patients?

A. For us, (we're Medicare, and we're expanding beyond Medicare) a home health aide would schedule five to seven patients a day. If all of them had a mental health diagnosis, seven patients would be too much. Patients with a psychiatric diagnosis will take longer, so it's harder for them. I set up the schedule according to the frequency of visits that the nurse and physician have decided upon. The home health aide schedules the time, goes to see the patient and she does do vital signs, and assists them with personal care, usually a bath. We have stretched it a little bit, depending on the needs, to retrain the patient, cuing them with cleaning their home, or doing the dishes, or going to the washroom, or making sure that they have the food they need in the home. We have extended our plan of care when a patient was agoraphobic by going for a walk— that was getting a little creative. We've had really good success where patients' homes were chaotic, or unlivable conditions, where we've had the psychiatric occupational therapist go in and do some clear cuing and work with the home health aide.

Q. Cuing is instruction?

A. Yes, a kind of instruction, saying this is the way you wash the dishes or prepare breakfast. They may have a medical or psychological diagnosis. They may be disabled.... It all depends on where they're at functionally. The most valuable experience we've had is where the psychiatric occupational therapist and the home health aide work together.

Q. And the psychiatric occupational therapist is a therapist?

A. An occupational therapist educated in the care of patients who cannot function.

Q. And it's up to the home health aide to call in the psychiatric occupational therapist?

A. Actually, it's usually the nurse who does that.

Q. How often does the nurse see the patient as opposed to the home health aide?

A. In a Medicare agency, the nurse has to be in there once every two weeks. Quite often a nurse may go into the home once or twice a week, while the home health aide could be in there two to three times a week. And our home health aides are very good at reporting any change in the patient's condition.

Q. If the condition is progressive, these people would be sent to a nursing home?

A. With us in there, home health aide giving some relief to the family and some support, we're often able to prevent nursing home placements; that's very important to us.

Q. Let's talk about earnings and career ladders?

A. I don't think they're part of a career ladder yet, though some of our CNAs [can be], if they get into a place that offers tuition reimbursement. I have three CNAs who are going to nursing school. Very often I have some single moms who are home health aides, too. As far as a career ladder, you can get additional training, but it doesn't mean you get additional pay. You can get rehab training, for example. There are some proposals by the National HomeCare Council to have some of those things, maybe levels of home health aides that would allow for reimbursement.

Q. I've seen a trend taking the jobs that can be done by nonclinical personnel and giving them to paraprofessionals, to free up the physicians and nurses.

A. They're wonderful. The educational level is different, but their ability to function given the right tools, communication, and reporting skills, are fine. But it's a group that also needs very strong supervision and support. Like I said, if I assigned five mental health patients to an aide in one day, I'd have to very carefully look for burnout.

I've seen high turnover rates, with the mental health worker, so it depends on the individual, how long they can work on this and how effective they can be.

Q. If you were advising someone, what could you tell them?

A. A high school person going into the field? It would depend on their situation. Getting nursing certification is a great start. You're dealing with basic human functions and that's what the reality of health care is. And it gives you a chance to see whether you're going to have the temperament. And it also gives you an idea of how things work, in the field, in the home, with the patients. I guess for a CNA entering the health care field, whether a nurse, therapist, or physician, it's an excellent way to get exposure to health care.

For people who come to me looking for jobs, I recommend that they get into a job that gives them some experience, and further their education so they can make some decent money, if that's where they need to be.

CAROLYN SCOTT, MS, RN, DIRECTOR

For more advanced nursing work as a home health aide, more training is advocated by professionals like registered nurse Carolyn Scott, who is the director of the Psychiatric Home Care Program, Rush Home Care Network. She discusses the range of jobs that will be needed in psychiatric home care. Notice how important medical nursing training is in combination with mental health skills.

Q. Your program has a specialty orientation, with academic and research areas cooperating on the clinical and practical side of medicine, and it sounds like your program is set up the same way. You've been going since 1988, so you know the field. What is happening in the field? Is it growing and changing to an outpatient emphasis?

A. Yes. It's growing. Absolutely. Our program was begun in 1988. We consider this a new specialty within home care. We're hospital-based, an academic facility, and we're listed under community health. We're considered community health nurses, but with a specialty in psychiatry.

It's considered one of the larger, more prestigious programs in the country. Most agencies are trying to become one-stop shopping agencies. They're trying to capture business and say they can do everything, total patient care through the life cycle, from birth through death. They would have all services, including psychiatric services. If you look at most of these areas in home care, at the needs of all the patients in home care, all of them have a psychosocial component that runs through their areas of care. So we've been conceptualizing a new "product line," as it's called. We have a health care team in psychiatry that will be able to handle all the needs of the psychiatric patient, and then if we need to bring in medical nurses, physical therapy, and so forth, we can do that. We have psychiatric occupational therapists and designated social workers who have special expertise in psychiatry. And we have home health aides who have had special in-service training in psychiatry, so if there were to be a new position created, like a mental health tech sort of person, they would be part of the health care team in psychiatry.

Q. What is the trend for education for those who are in Medicare/ mental health home care? Medicare has a lot to do with whom you can hire. Can you discuss the reasons for being so careful about psychiatric nurse requirements?

A. Most of our nurses come from an inpatient hospital background, and this requires as the base level of education, a B.S. in nursing. And then they took the registered nurse exam, so they have the credential of a registered nurse, and then they have the academic credential of a bachelor of science in nursing. We consider this a new specialty within home care; we're hospital based, and it's an academic facility so we're under community health nursing. The nurses are considered community health nurses, but with a specialty in psychiatry.

They had to get the psychiatric experience somewhere. Most of the nurses are currently master's prepared, which means they've taken two years of graduate education with clinical supervision in some outpatient treatment modality. I happened to do mine at a day hospital, some people do it in outpatient clinics. There are various situations where people can get that mental health experience and it's done with supervision. That's the model now. Social worker and psychologists do counseling.

The difference between psychiatric home care nurses and social workers is that social workers are not certified to work with medications and nurses are, and you're dealing with a lot of medications, because the treatment modality now is more psychopharmacology and biochemical treatment of the disorder. It is also a cost issue. Often, you're looking at someone who has a biochemical imbalance and it can be corrected with a medication. So it takes a certain high level of expertise to understand these patients.

Q. What is the best way to get into this field and get the necessary education?

A. At the very least, they need to get into a mental health career such as a mental health tech, but even inpatient hospitals won't hire high school graduates. I think the fastest-growing area is home health aide.

That would be the area I would turn them to. Those programs would develop special programs for home health aides who like to work with psychiatric patients.

Q. And to go beyond that into nursing? Is a master's necessary?

A. We're at a crossroads now. At the very least they'd need a bachelor's degree. I wouldn't go so far as to say they'd need a master's degree, but they'd have to take extra clinical rotations in school that would support mental health, be it psychology classes, chemistry, pharmacology, all the sciences—they would want to be at the very least a bachelor of science. For people who don't have very much money for that, they are bringing the LPNs back, licensed practical nurses. They are able to do very limited things. You would not have much room for advancement with that. They would have to go on for more education. You need people who have all of the equipment they need to keep their work as safe as possible.

Q. Is your mission to serve the indigent as well as the insured private-pay patient?

A. Yes, and soup to nuts. Medicare, public aid, and private insurance. And we're right now looking to get a managed care contract. I'm negotiating with the office of the public guardian for a contract. They have wards of the state. They're not all public aid. Many of them are very wealthy. We're trying to add on the nursing piece to their case management because they don't have a nurse; they have social work case managers.

Q. How many staff do you have? What does it take to run a county-wide operation?

A. Well I have two teams. In the Chicago office, I have six nurses full-time and three part-time. And then in the other office, I have two full-time and six part-time. And I guess we're doing around together maybe 10,000 to 13,000 visits a year.

Q. What might be the role of aides in the home health care of the future?

A. I can see a role for the high school student if we go into twenty-four-hour, seven-day crisis intervention triage and treatment in the private sector. Probably as a companion, someone would be there with the patient, to maintain safety, particularly if you're trying to monitor a patient in the home. Which is probably where we're going to be headed—maintaining them at home, one-to-one-ing them.

TRAINING FOR GERIATRIC HOME CARE

Through a government grant, two nurses, Joan Dreyfus, APRN, MSN, and Janice Gibeau, RN, Ph.D., developed an educational program especially aimed at home health care aides and geriatric care. They piloted the program at the University of Bridgeport, CT, and other colleges adopted it as well. It had a high mental health content.

In their book, *A Manual for Training Psychiatric Supportive Home Health Aides,* they described the health care challenge that's coming with the turn of the century. By the year 2030, sixty-six million Americans will be age sixty-five and older. As lifespans increase, there will be more frail elderly in need of care. Health care workers must cope with the following problems:

anxiety
difficult behavior
pain management
family dynamics
elder abuse
substance abuse and the elderly
paranoia and suspiciousness
dementia
dying and grief

In their curriculum, case histories taught students how to deal with these problems more effectively. Obviously, the more complex problems require professional medical attention. But the home health aide can cope with some of them. For instance, training and role-playing in the classroom can teach a home health aide how to defuse situations where a patient may be angry or combative. Health aides who may have never witnessed depression, dementia, or emotional illnesses are then ready for the realities of their fieldwork with patients. The chances are one in five that a senior will have some mental health element in his or her health care treatment. About 20 percent to as high as 50 percent of the medically ill elderly may have depressive symptoms. For all these reasons, the home health aide has a big responsibility. Most quality agencies develop standards for training and for behavior. For example, the Cleveland Clinic has a code for patient treatment that is a model for others:

1. Beneficence—do good to your patients.
2. Non-maleficence—do not harm your patients.
3. Freedom—invite your patients to participate in therapy.
4. Justice—distribute limited resources fairly.

Overcoming emotional problems and differing backgrounds can be challenging; it's an important part of the home health aide's job to learn to relate to all types of patients and treat them fairly. If the limited resources of the mental health system are to be used to their maximum, home health aides and other paraprofessional workers will have to play a role in the care of patients with medical and mental diagnoses.

Co-author Joan Dreyfus, APRN, MSN, explained some of the insights she gained from developing the geriatric mental health curriculum. She writes and teaches in addition to her career in group private practice with an agency, Geriatric Nursing Services.

Q. With the shift in the mental health workplace for the aging population from the traditional nursing home to group homes, assisted living, and residential settings, will there be more opportunities for home health aides and other workers?

A. I think there will be more opportunities. Anyone who's clinically involved in geriatrics, whether it's home care or partial or traditional nursing home, is aware that there's a big need for people on the home health aide level or even the companion level to have some training in psychiatric issues because so many of the elderly have a psychiatric overlay [psychiatric problems on top of medical ones], dementia being the major one. Now at this point, Medicare doesn't see that and doesn't pay anything extra, so there's no extra money for the training. Part of the goal of our grant was to demonstrate that you could do that and it wouldn't be too expensive. It was really an educational training grant from the AOA, the federal Agency on Aging.

Q. How did you become a certified nurse practitioner?

A. The hard way. I went through a three-year basic RN program back in the dark ages. Then I went back and got my bachelor's degree and I got my master's at Yale. That's a two-year clinical program. And I was working full-time all along, in various capacities.

Q. How did you finance your education?

A. I was lucky. I was doing my bachelor's during the era when if you were a nurse working full-time in a hospital, they were liberal with the tuition benefits. I actually got my bachelor's part-time in five years. I didn't pay a cent because the hospital where I worked full-time paid tuition. But then when I went to graduate school I had to go full-time and so I had to get loans. Yale was expensive, but not all that expensive.

Q. What training is necessary now to get into the field? For nurses?

A. There are several ways to go. There's still going the home health route, you get your training there from a home health agency; community colleges and hospitals or nursing homes have their own courses. Each state has standards you have to go by if you're going to do this. In Connecticut, it's a sixty-hour training program that people get to be certified home health aides. The state board of nursing or your community college may have the information.

Q. But make sure it's approved by the state before you enroll?

A. Yes. Now there are people who go through an associate degree program and get an associate degree program in geriatrics, counseling, or something like that. The other way to get into it would be to go the traditional routes of recreational therapy, occupational therapy, physical therapy, and nursing.

Q. I've heard that physical therapists are much in demand.

A. Yes. They can write their own ticket. I don't know how much longer that's going to last. Nurses were in the same situation a few years ago. Now nurses can still write their own ticket in home care, but not in hospitals.

And that would be another way to get into it. All of those positions usually have assistant levels that go along with them. You have a recreational therapy assistant, or an occupational therapy assistant, and usually the assistant is someone with an associate degree and little on-the-job training.

Q. Is there any pattern in the kind of people who go into the field?

A. Among the home health aides I've worked with, they're often sandwich-generation people who have older relatives or experience in taking care of older relatives. Also, these are people who are working to survive. They're often the breadwinners in their family and they work very hard.

There are other levels of occupations, too. In Connecticut, there's a job level we call homemaker. You work for an agency that supplies home health aides and companions and homemakers. And this is 98 percent for the elderly.

Q. What's the level of mental health involvement?

A. Well, with the geriatric home care that I'm doing now, one of the things I'm running into is that the homemaker is the cheapest person to put into the home and they're often put in it with the severe Alzheimer's patient and don't know what to do. It's not their fault; they've never had any training. Home health aides also have difficulty if they don't have adequate training. Agencies are looking for the least expensive level and that's one of the dilemmas. Some patients don't fit the Medicaid criteria for skilled care. They don't need somebody to change their colostomy dressing, or even take their blood pressure. They need help with getting dressed and not burning themselves on the stove. That's not considered skilled by the reimbursement agencies. And so they get this level of care from a person who usually has no training and it doesn't work very well unless you happen to luck into someone who has had this experience in life.

Q. Do you see changes with the increases in aging population?

A. I see signs they will be cutting now in New York state.

Q. But is this an entry point into the field, a place to start?

A. Yes that's true. And you do have people who go on, to the two-year RN program. There used to be LPNs, but they're pretty much extinct around here.... If you don't have the certification behind you of being a social worker or a nurse or a physical therapist, it's very hard to get jobs. The people who run agencies for the elderly are driven by Medicare, and if Medicare doesn't have a slot that's going to pay your job description, they're not going to be able to pay you. You can get a degree in counseling and work as a companion or a homemaker, but people tend not to like to do that. People go to college and they think they should do something better. It's difficult with just those general kinds of counseling degrees.

With a wide range of jobs and skill levels to choose from, home health will be a promising field for many job seekers during the coming five to ten years. Although, like some of the people interviewed here, you may begin in a hospital setting, the opportunities of the future may lead you to consider home health agencies as well.

FOR MORE INFORMATION

American Hospital Association
    Division of Nursing
    1 North Franklin
    Chicago, IL 60661

    For information about nursing aides and psychiatric aides.

Foundation for Hospice and Homecare
    519 C Street NE
    Stanton PK
    Washington, DC 20002

    This group offers a national homemaker-home health aide certification. Includes the former National HomeCaring Council.

American Nurses' Association
    600 Maryland Avenue SW
    Washington, DC 20024-2571

Visiting Nurses Association of America
    3801 East Florida, Suite 900
    Denver, CO 80210-2545

CHAPTER 5

CRISIS MANAGEMENT

On the front lines of mental health work are crisis intervention workers. At a community agency, a hospital, or a welfare agency, these workers are ready to respond to an emergency situation. Much of the work is done by telephone. A typical first contact with a distressed person is a call to a crisis intervention worker answering a twenty-four-hour phone line. Crisis workers have to be ready for all kinds of calls, from people who may just be lonely or from a despondent caller who's suicidal. Because of the volume of calls, these hotlines need volunteers and/or paraprofessionals. A good crisis center will train its phone workers to screen calls and will make provision to transfer serious calls to trained psychiatrists who deal with the most difficult problems.

Typical job titles may be:

case management aide
social work assistant
community outreach worker
crisis intervention worker
crisis prevention worker

After the initial call, a counselor may take over, screening the call and assessing the caller's problem, then discussing it within the crisis agency's own staff.

The community mental health center movement in the sixties and seventies envisioned a crisis center as a hub in a network of services. This system placed nonprofessionals in the position of providing timely help for foreseeable life crises and accidental crises. "A little help at the right time is more preventive than long-term help," wrote Francine

Sobey in her 1970 book, *The Nonprofessional Revolution in Mental Health.* It was clear that the number of psychiatrists was too small to provide advanced professional help to everyone in every community. The introduction of paraprofessionals as crisis workers could expand the reach of the community centers.

Did the idea work? One answer is seen in the large number of crisis lines in any big city in the country today. In the Chicago area, the crisis lines are the first link in a network of social services. Crisis lines cover many special problems: for instance, in the metropolitan area there are five crisis lines for abuse—domestic, child, or spouse abuse. Some are run by private agencies, others are public mental health agency projects. Alcoholism/drug abuse crisis lines often connect with local hospitals; seven out of eleven crisis lines in Chicago go to hospital-based services, reflecting the need for inpatient or outpatient treatment for people who have these kinds of problems. Family support crisis lines abound, and people in need can be referred to psychiatric help, food, shelter, parental counseling, and other forms of assistance via these connections. Services with terminal connections for the hearing impaired also are important, providing TTY/TDD connections for electronic devices that allow the deaf to communicate via keyboard with helpers at crisis centers.

Multiple outlets in the city serve the homeless with telephone helplines for emergency services. With about 25 to 30 percent of the homeless classified as having a mental diagnosis of some kind, these can be a vital link with social services and the indigent mentally ill population.

Crisis centers come in all types and sizes. Experience has shown the value of setting up crisis lines and drop-in centers to help people deal with their problems and the value of trained nonprofessionals to staff those phone lines.

Crisis centers such as those run by the Red Cross also react when there's been a natural disaster, a flood for example, that has left victims traumatized. While physicians can treat their physical scars, who will treat the psychological scars, and who will help the victims regain a normal life? Mental health services such as counseling are recognized as a part of the healing process in these situations.

A community may be affected by a high-stress situation, such as the closing of a plant, resulting in layoffs of hundreds of workers, many of them family breadwinners. A natural disaster can create severe stress, requiring follow-up by local and state mental health professionals. Sometimes work can go on for years afterward, as unmet needs are recognized and attended to. For example, following the Midwest floods of 1993, considerable efforts by the Bi-State Red Cross and county and state officials in Missouri continued well into 1995. The Red Cross provided mental health services in the form of trained Red Cross counselors and community volunteers who helped victims cope with the disaster. The St. Louis Bi-State Chapter of the Red Cross recorded 16,910 mental health contacts in eastern Missouri and southern Illinois during 1993. Displaced persons required housing. Families had lost their life savings, possessions, and property. They required counseling by social workers. Children who'd lost their homes and were uprooted from their communities were offered counseling. A long-term assistance program was developed by public and private agencies, including the United Way, to address problems of disabilities, unemployment, and impoverishment.

To be involved in this kind of work, contact public agencies such as county emergency management departments, mental health departments, and private social services agencies. Training appropriate for emergency services is similar to human services and social work education.

Particular interests within the mental health field will determine an appropriate course of study. There are numerous certificate and associate degree programs that offer human services or mental health majors. Some 375 such programs were counted in 1992 by the federal government; they are located at community and junior colleges, vocational-technical institutes, and other schools. (See Chapter 7 on human services for a sample of the curriculum for an associate degree in mental health technology or human services.) Beyond these degree programs, 390 programs provide a bachelor's degree in human services. Some programs include courses in crisis intervention—look for these if this is the specialty you want. You'll also study psychology, social work, family dynamics, rehabilitation, and other subjects. Not only will you attend classes, you'll also engage in simulations, role-playing, and other learning techniques that prepare you for real situations you'll encounter in the working world. In certificate programs, you may do fieldwork with clinical supervision.

FLORENCE FORSHEY, COMMUNITY
CENTER SUPERVISOR

Still more in need of mental health care are the victims of domestic violence. Florence Forshey runs the Des Plaines Valley Community Center. One of its specialties is domestic violence. One focus of the center is a program for battered women. Workers help women recover from abuse and assault. They provide medical assistance in cooperation with local hospitals. They offer help with legal remedies that take women and their children out of dangerous domestic situations where they have been physically abused, and put them on the road to recovery.

Another service offered at the Des Plaines center is substance abuse counseling. The problems of substance abuse and domestic violence can be interrelated. If one or both spouses are chemically dependent, and the husband is abusive, the situation is all the worse. Their families may have to separate themselves from the abusive family member. For those who are dependent on drugs and who become violent, counseling is often the best way to begin to break the cycle and return to reality—if they can be persuaded to enter counseling. Even though dependence may be psychological and the use of violence unnecessary, it can be difficult if not impossible for habitual offenders to quit without the help that trained professionals can offer. However, the first duty of society is to get the endangered family members to safety. Florence Forshey's program does that. In an interview, she explains what kinds of workers are hired, how they're trained, and tells what it's like to work there. Some of the following material is disturbing, but it is not unrepresentative of the situations that crisis workers may encounter.

Q. What kind of employees work with you at entry-level jobs? What kind of work goes on at the center?

A. We train students from University of Illinois, the University of Chicago, and the junior colleges. An AA (associate) degree worker is occasionally hired for the shelter. If they want to move up, workers have to go on and get more education. We've had people as community workers with not even an AA degree when we had an intake worker position.

People would come in with unpaid bills, eviction notices, and we would help with those kinds of services which are very important to them. The problem for centers like ours is that funding is not matching needs. When funding gets tight, you begin to make choices. In the areas of dual diagnosis, such as a combined mental health and addiction diagnosis, people need a lot of concrete support. We service about 500 to 600 a year in addictions; and in our domestic violence program, we serve about 1,200; so we'll see 2,000 to 2,500 in a year total.

Q. What's the ranger of entry-level jobs with a mental health care component in the job setting?

A. In domestic violence counseling, the minimum is usually a B.A. in human services. I don't like it when we hire people without B.A.s, although we do sometimes. We don't have the luxury of hiring many assistants; our salaries are low. State funding is scarce but is one of our major sources.

In mental health there are two entry-level positions here. One provides education and the other does court appearances with clients. Court advocates at the Des Plaines Valley Center are intermediaries between the domestic violence survivor and the court. If a woman comes into the shelter for assistance, we help her to see what options are available. She's usually been abused by a husband or boyfriend, left him, and sought protection or help. Also at entry-level are children's counselors. B.A.-level education is standard. These people have to be trained to work with children who've been assaulted. These counselors are assigned to provide support under the direction of social work supervisors, and they also have to be prepared to work with the depressed, schizoid, etc. A psychiatrist comes in to monitor medications for the clients.

We have a public mental health agency whose job is to be a liaison with Madden Mental Health Center and with our hospitals in the area: Loyola, Hines, Madden. We see 500 people in the mental health unit a year. There's a large sexual assault unit in the center. This is one of the few social service agencies working with children and women who've been assaulted.

Q. What training do you recommend for people who want to work at a center like yours?

A. I believe that a college education is needed. A B.A. is recommended. These workers need interview skills and a sense of themselves. They usually have had two courses in developmental psychology and already have an understanding of mental illness problems. They should have had some exposure to working with a population of assault victims. In an entry-level position, you help a woman get through the maze of the court system.

Q. What other services are offered at the center?

A. Another service of the center is substance abuse. In substance abuse again, my salaries are low. The job situation is different in substance abuse. We were looking for Hispanic addictions counselors, and there were only twelve in the state (ten years ago.) Many counselors were recovering abusers. Now there are courses; almost everyone has a B.A.; some have M.A.s. One is a master's-level social worker. That person just graduated recently but was working here for years and got her education during the time she was working here. So, she has a combination of experience and education.

Q. What are the working conditions in the center? What is a typical workweek?

A. The mental health unit is open fifty-five hours a week. The addictions unit is open fifty-nine hours a week. There's flexibility in the shifts.

Q. How can you advance after starting to work at a center?

A. People who work with us and go on to get a degree can go on in the field much more easily. A lot of our staff have stayed with us a long time. We offer flexibility of hours. At the addiction center, a woman worker had a B.A., was interested in addiction, and got certification as an addiction counselor (CAC), and came back to us from Grant (Grant Hospital, Chicago) after a two-year course. One woman has become an expert and has worked with sexually assaulted children.

Q. What are typical earnings of the people who work at the center?

A. Salaries for addictions workers start below $20,000. Mental health salaries start low, but we have a commitment to pay them at $18,000–$19,000. Until a few years ago, pay was $16,000 for a B.A.; we now try to pay more in the domestic violence area. We have had difficulty in state funding, static or regressive. I lost 21 percent of funding in the adolescent unit; 5 percent in domestic violence unit.

Q. Why is there the emphasis on domestic violence and substance abuse, versus other services?

A. There is a need for our services. Our waiting list in addictions has been as high as 100. With the new criteria for addictions, managed care

model, we're finding we have to see people rapidly. It's made it difficult. People don't stay as long for treatment.

In a center of this type, with multiple services, there are usually a few
entry-level positions that need to be filled. Large hospitals and other major health care facilities need many mental health workers, but if you prefer community mental health care, you may find that there are only one
or two entry-level jobs at each center. They require a person with some
training, ideally some course work in psychology. Workers who started
their careers as assistants at the center took additional course work during their off-hours. While they worked, they continued their education
and moved up to social workers, domestic violence counselors, or substance abuse counselors at the center or other facilities like it.

A trend in crisis intervention identified recently by *Hospitals* magazine involves emergency department (ED) social workers at hospitals.
These ED social workers take over the tasks of helping patients' families arrange for home health care or nursing home beds, if needed. They
help direct patient traffic to the right place, so that ED physicians and
nurses can work on the true emergencies. The hospital can avoid unnecessary admissions, and the patients are better served as a result.

A smaller hospital that started this program is Miami Valley Medical
Center in Ohio. The idea spread and many emergency units may have
social workers attached to them. Duke University Medical Center,
Durham, NC, is one example of a large hospital that has the capacity to
support this level of mental health care.

Crisis prevention workers have a different role. These workers help
people to stay out of the kind of trouble that the crisis intervention workers must deal with. They work in neighborhood centers and make themselves available to all persons in their territory or "cachement area."

The skills needed for crisis work vary. A hotline worker may be a volunteer or a part-time worker trained to screen calls and thus has little
formal education. However, this or her supervisors may be degreed
counselors. The worker may give out basic advice for the current crisis
or arrange for assistance by counselors at a later time.

Advance workers have all the skills associated with counseling and
psychiatry. Programs now exist that train social workers at the graduate
level in crisis intervention.

The discontentments that accompany daily life occasionally break out into violence. These incidents have occurred in many cities, when mentally disturbed individuals become violent. Then, crisis workers are needed to deal with a problem that can affect an entire community. An incident need not even involve violence to create a traumatic situation where counseling professionals could be of help. For example, a death of a well-known student at a local high school in an auto accident, or the suicide of a youth, may be cause to call in outside help to assist those in the school in dealing with their grief.

Then, too, the modern plague of AIDS has created difficult situations for sufferers of the disease. Once diagnosed as HIV positive, an individual may have ongoing need for help in a variety of areas, not just medical, but psychological, employment, and other types of assistance.

There are many situations where crisis intervention is necessary. It takes a special type of person to assist those in need. The first contact is important, but follow-up is even more so. Crisis agencies have plans for referrals to the kinds of professionals who can assist their client population. Examples are social workers, psychiatrists, and visiting nurses. The whole range of community services may be needed at different times with various types of callers.

Working in a crisis center can be a good start, even if you are volunteering while still a student. Many crisis centers need part-time workers. If you begin to work at such a place while you're still in school, you'll find out if you like the feeling of helping people there and you can get the experience it takes to begin building up a resume, and perhaps qualify for scholarships to continue your education in human services or social work.

FOR MORE INFORMATION

National Association of Social Workers
  750 First Street NE
  Suite 700
  Washington, DC 20002–4241

Council on Social Work Education
    1600 Duke Street
    Alexandria, VA 22314-3421

    An annual directory of accredited B.S.W. and M.S.W. programs is available for $10.

National Organization for Human Service Education
    Brookdale Community College
    Lyncroft, NJ 07738

American Red Cross
    National Headquarters
    430 Seventeenth Street NW
    Washington, DC 20006-2800

United Way of America
    701 North Fairfax Street
    Alexandria, VA 22314-2045

CHAPTER 6

SUBSTANCE ABUSE AND CHEMICAL DEPENDENCY

Perhaps no other area of mental health care has touched as many families and individuals in America as drug and alcohol abuse treatment. Constantly we are warned against drunk driving, drug abuse, and the host of ills that accompany these habits. Addiction, whether physical or psychological, or chemical dependency on drugs or alcohol, has afflicted millions. According to the National Clearinghouse for Alcohol and Drug Information, 10 million Americans are alcoholics; another 7 million abuse alcohol. Police arrest 1.4 million people for drunk driving and auto fatalities involving alcohol number 25,000 a year now. Some 95,000 deaths due to alcoholism occurred in 1985. Drugs, too, are widespread as 20 million people use marijuana, 22.7 million have used cocaine at least once, and 3 million have used crack. Not everyone develops a habitual or addictive use of a drug. Although 100 million people drink, only 10 percent of them suffer from alcoholism. Still, the consequences are grave for those who become dependent. As a result, an enormous need has developed for professionals who can cope with the consequences in lost productivity, suffering, physical and psychological illness, and violence.

Alcohol abuse is a problem of long standing. From Alcoholics Anonymous (AA) to the hospital-based detoxification units that treat patients, a wide variety of treatments are available. Most involve a step-by-step program of treatment, based often on AA's twelve-step program that begins with the confession that the individual has a problem and leads to abstinence from alcohol (and/or drugs). The accepted medical theory now is that alcoholism and substance abuse are diseases, and that there may be a genetic component that makes some people more likely to become dependent.

Treatment requires medical attention. Detoxification may take place in a hospital, followed by outpatient treatment in other settings like halfway houses, support groups of other ex-drinkers, and visits to rehabilitation programs. An alcoholism counselor may lead the program, or the health care professional may be a psychologist or psychiatrist. Alcoholics Anonymous has proven to be successful with peer groups of ex-drinkers helping each other.

Alcoholism is also a mental health problem. Both alcoholics and drug abusers are likely to be out of touch with reality. They may be suicidal in some cases. The reasons for their dependence may have psychological sources in personality problems. So, it's believed that full treatment of the disease should address these underlying causes.

Drug abuse is a newer problem in America, but one that has become more pervasive. Although America briefly adopted a permissive attitude to drugs in the 1960s, the consensus developed that there could be no tolerance for drug abuse. Government and private programs sought to remedy the problem. However, more drugs are being added to the list of those commonly abused, and not only soft drugs like marijuana but cocaine, crack, and others have become well known. Complicating the drug problem is the drug culture and the underground economy it has spawned—drug sales and eventually drug wars among rival dealers and the police. Central to the problem is the youth of many of the users. Teens have become involved in drug experimentation in great numbers, and more than a third of all teens used illicit drugs in 1979; in 1991 a fifth of teens were estimated to have tried drugs; nearly half had tried alcohol.

Health care providers sought to help. Some programs were preventive in nature, such as the "Just Say No" commercial campaigns sponsored by government and health groups. Some sought to deal with the reality of the situation, helping drug users with their problems, as the Haight Ashbury Clinic in San Francisco did beginning in the psychedelic years of the 1960s. New York City, after considerable controversy, began a program of dispensing clean needles to addicts to prevent HIV infection. Many community agencies developed drug hotlines to deal with

Alcohol and Drug Abuse

(Percent of total U.S. population age 12 and up)

	Any illicit drug	*Marijuana*	*Cocaine*	*Alcohol*	*Cigarettes*
Total	37.2	33.7	11.3	83.6	71.2
Male	42.4	39.2	14.5	87.8	76.6
Female	32.4	28.7	8.5	79.8	66.3

(Percent of teens age 12–17 who have ever used)

	Any illicit drug	*Marijuana*	*Cocaine*	*Alcohol*	*Cigarettes*
Total	17.9	11.7	1.1	41.3	34.5
Male	17.8	12.7	0.9	40.7	34.0
Female	18.0	10.6	1.4	42.1	35.0

Source: National Household Survey on Drug Abuse: Population Estimates, 1993. Substance Abuse and Mental Health Services Administration, Office of Applied Studies, U.S. Department of Health and Human Services, U.S. Public Health Service.

overdose situations and to encourage users who wanted to quit. Many of these services were good training grounds for volunteers and paraprofessional mental health workers.

A variety of treatments in appropriate settings is needed. Hospitals treat the most seriously affected. For example, a cocaine overdose can be life-threatening, or a drug abuser can intentionally alter his or her mental state. Habitual users may have serious personal problems that lead them to try to escape the reality of their daily life through drugs. Hospitalization may be needed for a few days to detoxify them and make sure the drug is no longer affecting them. Later, they may need counseling if they are suicidal, depressed, or have other problems that relate to mental illness. That's where drug abuse counselors can help by assisting them to deal with the real problems after they give up drugs. Physicians have found that many people who abuse drugs also abuse alcohol; they call this co-addiction. The extended use of the addictive drugs and drink may change a person's behavior, or exaggerate problems they have already, and lead to panic disorders, anxiety, and antisocial personality disorders. The drug abuse counselor has to sort out the problems and assess the person's reasons for doing drugs and the effects the drugs have had.

After a crisis is over, the effects of chemical dependency, which lead to a psychological addiction, still remain and need to be addressed. An example of a center that did just that was the Irene Whitney Center in Minneapolis, the "first halfway house for chemically dependent teenagers and young adults," which operated continuously from 1976 to 1992. Long-term treatment of some kind may be helpful. Halfway houses can deal with patients' needs.

Some evidence shows that such treatment has been successful long-term, as prevention efforts have been. In 1990, 48 percent of high school seniors had used an illicit drug at least once, according to *American Demographics* magazine. In 1980, 66 percent had. That's progress, but problems still exist. Some experimenters become regular users. There's an ongoing need to treat those for whom drugs become a problem.

Indeed, the latest surveys tend to show that teens aren't as convinced of the dangers of drug use as they once were. The "Monitoring the Future" study by the University of Michigan's Institute for Social Research tracked a resurgence of marijuana use since 1991, after a turnaround in the drug use epidemic of that late 1970s and a decline until 1992. For these reasons, opportunities abound for workers in drug and alcohol treatment. Former users are valuable workers in the drug abuse programs of many cities. Those who are streetwise and experienced can give recovering patients some insights about getting off and staying off drugs. Because the problem is so pervasive, there is a need almost everywhere for workers to cope with the influx of people seeking treatment.

If you're a drug abuse worker, you may work a phone hotline, answering calls from the public. Hotline staffers may call a hospital ER for a drug overdose or calm down a frightened youth enduring a bad drug experience. You may work in the intake unit of a drug abuse program, signing up new people. You will help drug counselors work to change the personality that has become dependent on a drug.

Drug programs take many forms and are found in many settings, from education programs to community center crisis programs to hospital emergency or inpatient treatment. Training in crisis counseling can be valuable.

Drug abuse workers may also need expertise in pharmacology. Working in a substance abuse program can be a good start for a mental health career. Many of these programs are well funded and innovative. They need your help as a worker. The entry-level position may be called substance abuse technician or intake aide, depending on the agency. Educational requirements vary. Often, a former drug user who's recovering finds a job with a substance abuse program. Supervisors, though, tend to be psychologists or counselors with advanced training. The treatment philosophy may differ from agency to agency, though many adopt AA's twelve-step program while others prefer what's called "rational recovery" or some other method. The AA methods were extended to drug abusers through Narcotics Anonymous and Cocaine Anonymous. In any system, it's a major time commitment for patients. Here's a description of one program in the Chicago area through an interview with its director.

DON NEITZEL, DIRECTOR, PARKSIDE RECOVERY

Q. What's your role as director here at Parkside Recovery? What's your mission?

A. Interestingly I've been with Parkside for six years and I've been in various roles, director of marketing and community relations and now the director of behavioral medicine for the hospital. I really didn't get involved too heavily in clinical work. However, for ten years I was the co-director of the outpatient program. What has guided me throughout the period of time have been the principles of Alcoholics Anonymous.

Q. I notice the mission statement refers to addiction treatment. What is included in that category?

A. Our focus is on addiction to chemicals. We don't have a primary food disorder program or a primary gambling program or anything of that nature. We have an addictions unit and a psychiatric unit. Parkside manages both of them through me. My background basically has been addictions as opposed to the psychiatric field. However, administratively, the requisite is not an in-depth knowledge of psychiatry; it is the ability to manage people.

Q. Could you tell me something about the staff itself? You mentioned counselors. What other personnel do you require?

A. During the daytime, three full-time nurses, two substance abuse technicians, and a unit secretary on the inpatient unit. On the outpatient unit there's the admissions team, a coordinator, two admissions specialists, and a secretary. And then we have three addictions counselors in the outpatient department.

Q. Parkside and the hospital share responsibility for the substance abuse program here?

A. I'm making some changes. We're transferring personnel. The majority of the personnel have been employed by Parkside. And this unit has been here since 1989. The hospital wants to assume more direct control over the employees, so with the exception of the administrative staff, the majority of the counselors are being transferred to and employed by Little Company of Mary Hospital [where the recovery program is located].

Q. How has substance abuse treatment changed in recent years?

A. In the eighties, managed care began to impact on the length of stays, so hospitals couldn't maintain an inpatient census over a protracted period of time. Stays were reduced from 25, 23, 22 days to 7, 6, or 5.

Q. What's the structure of management here and at the other Parkside units around the country?

A. There are fourteen in host hospitals around the country where the management, the administrative director, and generally a community relations or marketing person are the only Parkside employees at the facility. Parkside provides the clinical expertise and updating with current Joint Commission regulations, and formulating programs and things of that type, providing them for the hospital.

Q. Within this unit of Parkside, what do the technicians, counselors, and the nurses do?

A. At the technician level, there's the admissions specialist, who responds to inquiries about treatment, recovery, and substance abuse, and coordinates a smooth and responsive admission and referral process, and provides education for people who are chemically dependent and their families. Qualifications would include phone skills, typing skills, knowledge of alcoholism/substance abuse. Education requirements used to be an associate's degree in occupational therapy, but a bachelor's degree in social services is preferred now, along with certification in addiction counseling.

Q. There are two levels of counselors. The counselor IIs are master's level?

A. Yes. The counselor IIs are master's level. The addictions counselor I, under clinical supervision, provides counseling and program treatment to patients and families who have alcoholism and other chemical addictions, orients patients and their families to the treatment program, and encourages their active participation. The counselor has responsibility for an assigned caseload of patients: interviews, evaluates, and develops treatment plans for patients with approval of the program manager; prepares discharge and referral summaries; and documents all care in the patient record. The counselor has to conduct individual and group counseling and family and employer orientation counseling sessions. The counselor is an active team member in reviewing the patients' responses to the treatment program and recommending modifications to the treatment plans. The counselor presents information on treatment concepts, objectives, and goals to patients, their families, and friends. Counselors also observe patients' responses to treatment. Counselors work closely with referral sources. They have a working knowledge of AA and other twelve-step groups.

The qualifications for counselors are that they must be a graduate of a recognized twelve-month clinical counselor training program or the equivalent training. They are to be certified or eligible for certification as an alcoholism counselor. A bachelor's degree is preferred. If they're recovering, they must be active in AA/NA (Narcotics Anonymous) and must have four years' continuous abstinence if they were substance abusers.

Q. Is this staff inclusion of recovering people typical?

A. Historically it has been more unique to Parkside than other units.

Q. What makes a person decide to become a counselor?

A. For the most part I think for a recovering person I would say the motivation would be an extension of the philosophy that got them sober.

That they wanted to help other people. They wanted to be in the helping field, and since addiction was something that was personally known to them, it might be something they could impart and help other people with. With nonrecovering people, it might be someone in their history or something in their life experience; a problem they felt they could help with or wanted to be involved with.

Q. I wanted to come back to the technician's job. That sounds like an entry-level job. Does every recovery unit require someone like this?

A. Yes. Well admissions, for example, require about an hour and a half on the part of the treatment team. You have to get a nursing assessment, there are some release of information forms that need to be signed, some consent for treatment, some demographic data, all these things, so substance abuse technicians help with the admissions process. They will be involved with presentation of videos to patients, recreational activities, and a variety of things that would occur through the day.

Q. Is it possible to move up from there? To get education to be a counselor?

A. Yes. But that's a whole different thing. There would be a course of formal education that you would need. You would meet some minimum requirements that are part of the core of what you need for counselor training, do a six-month internship much like a master's-level person. These standards were devised by Parkside when they had three 100-bed units in Chicago when they could utilize ten to twelve counselor trainees a year.

Q. In addition to education, what would you look for in a person who's seeking to become a counselor?

A. Some exposure to a twelve-step program—whether AA or Alateen—so they can understand from a philosophical standpoint where we're coming from. Because our addiction model is utilization of a twelve-step support system when a person finishes treatment.

Q. As I understand it the twelve-step program involves recognition of the problem first and then of the need for help—that I need to stop drinking or abusing drugs, and I need to get help from somebody, more than what I can do for myself.

A. And recognition of a higher power. There are a few other methods, such as rational recovery, that are being implemented, however we don't subscribe to those. Our experience has taught us what has worked best for most has been AA and NA and CA (Cocaine Anonymous).

Q. Take me through a case history. If I came in and said—I've been having trouble, I'm drinking too much, I can't hold a job, I use drugs for escape and for my problems—what would I do, how would you help me?

A. I would assess the severity of usage. If a guy has a history of a usage of once or twice a week, the need for an inpatient setting doesn't exist. However, if there's a degree of unmanageability about his lifestyle, then he needs structure-building techniques that would allow him to make his life more manageable.

Q. Who would I encounter along the path of treatment?

A. You make a call to a facility. We schedule an evaluation, and depending on what is obtained in the results of the evaluation, we will make a recommendation for some level of treatment. Now, what would indicate that? The severity of dysfunction would be a contributing factor to inpatient or outpatient treatment, along with the physical complications that go along with substance abuse and the amount of current distress that the person's experiencing.

Some drugs by necessity would require an inpatient setting. Daily heroin use, for example, the detoxification process for heroin, as an aid to that a significant amount of medical management is required, and it's best done in an inpatient setting.

Q. I guess one of my stereotypes is the skidrow alcoholic, but there are also high-society alcoholics?

A. Yes, the "functional" and the whole spectrum of people around them, the family, who are drawn into the problem with them.

Q. Is that true of drug use, too?

A. Yes, of course, It's difficult to make a generic classification that "this guy's a cokehead" and envision that this is an unemployed person who's dysfunctional. I would say on a daily basis, we probably have sixty-five people in our facility, between inpatient and outpatient, somewhere between 80 and 90 percent are employed, so it's not a chronic skidrow person that you'd encounter. It's a very functional employed person that we have within our treatment center.

Q. What leads a person to this? Is it recreational use? Many people try it and stop. Some people go on and get addicted. What are the reasons?

A. Is there a genetic complication? Possibly. History has taught me that continued use of any drug, I don't care if there's predisposition, creates addiction. And with alcoholism or addiction to a sleeping pill or anything like that, there is an alteration in tolerance that occurs after significant use over a period of time. It's a chemical reaction. The dose has little or no effect so they increase the dose. So it's a progression. Do some people' personalities indicate that they're prone to addiction? I would say so. Does that mean it's a mental problem? I don't think so. I think addiction is a biochemical reaction to a drug.

Q. Can every addict recover?

A. My feeling is yes. Otherwise I wouldn't be in this field. I do think there is a possibility that they can recover. There are some that are essentially incapable of what is required in terms of honesty to recover.

Q. How important is a faith component? In other words, I believe in God, and I pray to God to get me out of this addiction.

A. Sometimes it has an effect, and I'm not going to discount it because many people have begun the road to recovery through religious fervor. Religion itself has no part, I don't think, in twelve-step recovery. Because the two are different. The spirituality that exist within the structure of AA or NA is not the spirituality that exists in the structure of a formalized religion.

Q. That power could come from the group?

A. Exactly.

Q. What would you say is the future in addiction treatment? Are we on the way to solving the problem? Or is this a growing problem that will require more professionals in the field to deal with it?

A. Do I think the problems are going to go away? No. Unless they stop making grapes, and they stop making cocoa leaves, and they stop making opium, poppies, whatever, I don't think it's going to go away. There are certainly going to be people who want for whatever reason to alter reality. And they will find whatever means are necessary—whether it's a grown product or a synthesized product—to alter their perception;

they're going to do it. Now, does education about addiction help? Yes. There's no doubt about it. That's one of the elements that occurs within the treatment setting no matter where you go, you get some basis of understanding of the progression of addiction. It becomes the obligation of the person who is in treatment to look at that and make a decision that this is correct information. Then make a decision based on what I have seen that this is applicable to me, "If I continue to use these bad things, I'm going to continue to have them." I think what occurs unfortunately is that many people begin to believe that they're impervious to the consequences of any kind of drug use, for whatever reason.

Do I think there's a future? Yes, I think there is. This hospital has made a decision to maintain an addictions unit in the hospital because they feel that it's an integral part of A. hospital admissions, and B. the wellness that needs to occur in the community in terms of treating illnesses. Now, does the setting change from what we have historically known as an inpatient setting to an outpatient setting? Yes, I think it will.

Q. OK, and there's a different set of personnel that you need for that?

A. There's an additional group that you need, but you also eliminate some. Nursing is reduced. The need for direct nursing care for outpatient for the most part is reduced to zero. Medical management, the stability of the patient, does not have to be managed on an ongoing basis.

Q. I suppose there'll still be some patients who require inpatient detoxification?

A. Absolutely. And a number of facilities have gone to excluding any inpatient setting and just having a small detoxification unit and the only treatment programs they provide are outpatient.

Q. Any advice you would give to people who are looking at the field, thinking they might want to find a career? What preparation would you suggest?

A. From a preparation standpoint, however many courses in addiction and psychology they can acquire from a formal education would certainly be beneficial. A number of the colleges in the area [Chicago] offer addiction-specific programs that would certainly be a plus to get into entry-level position. Most of them, at the completion of the required basic curriculum, offer the possibility of taking the certification exam for a counselor position. That credential would provide them with entrée into the field.

STANDARDS FOR PROGRAMS

Alcohol and drug treatment programs will be a part of most managed mental health programs in the future. Paraprofessionals will be needed both in prevention programs and in treatment programs in various capacities. Twelve-step programs need counselors to assist participants. New treatment methods such as naltrexone medication for detoxification treatment of alcoholism, may advance the process of recovery, but full recovery will probably still require monitoring by substance abuse workers, along with an overall program of counseling, education, and support.

There are many standards for programs treating alcoholism and for other drug dependence services, administered by the Joint Commission on Accreditation of Health Care Organizations. If you go to work in an alcohol or drug abuse program, you may be interested to know what a typical program must do to meet the standards of a quality-conscious accrediting body like the Joint Commission on Accreditation of Health Care Organizations. Good, accredited programs have the following features:

Good individualized treatment. The patient may have both a substance abuse diagnosis and mental disorder, so the program or service should be ready to manage both of these health problems. The program starts by investigating what caused the condition and what are its effects, on a "biopsychosocial" basis. The program should have a good system for handling patient referrals and documenting them. (That requires good intake workers.)

Good recovery programs that treat the special needs of children and teens. These include education, family, and development (biopsychosocial); effects of minor's legal status; nutrition; and recreational activities.

Knowledgeable and committed staff. Those who work with the drug-dependent patient need to be able to interview him or her to get information about the condition and be able to analyze that information about the dependence. They have to understand the conditions and environment that are affecting the patient's dependence. They also need to know how to get the patient the treatment that's needed, based on the available services.

Assessment of the patient. Assessing the patient starts with taking a history of the patient's use of alcohol and/or drugs. A physical health assessment is one part of this; emotional and behavioral factors also must be assessed. Medical personnel do the tests needed and the physical exams that test for dependence, disease, or physical abuse. Mental health professionals look into the emotional effects of the drug dependence on the patient, his or her memory, behavior, danger to himself or herself or others, and also the general mental condition.

Examination of family history. The service should also find out whether there's a family history of alcoholism or drug dependence. They need to know about education and job history. There's a need to examine the family and other relationships, daily activities, and influences on the patient such as values, beliefs, and spiritual orientation. All of this information should be summarized.

Since the seventies, nonprofessionals have helped drug and alcoholism programs in actual treatment. These techniques are directed to motivating patients to quit drinking using behavior modification. By reinforcing correct behavior, the staffs of these programs help their clients to return to normal life.

METHODS OF TREATMENT

Since paraprofessionals are active in the intake of patients, they need to be familiar with the methods of treatment. Of course, treatment of dependent people will be up to medical personnel and psychiatric clinicians.

The next ten years will see many changes in the requirements to become a drug abuse and alcoholism counselor. More states will require licensure; additional education will be more important for career advancement.

FOR MORE INFORMATION

National Association of Alcoholism and Drug Abuse Counselors
3717 Columbia Pike, Suite 300
Arlington, VA 22204-4254

Provides counselors with training and education resources, represents the interests of the profession, and offers information on becoming a counselor.

National Association of State Alcohol and Drug Abuse Directors
444 North Capital Street NW
Suite 642
Washington, DC 20001

National Clearinghouse for Alcohol and Drug Information (NCADI)
P.O. Box 2345
Rockville, MD 20852
800–729–6686

Information on research and statistics about alcohol and drug abuse.

National Institute of Drug Abuse and Confidential Referral Service
800–662–HELP

A publicly funded, free telephone service.

National Nurses Society on Addictions
4101 Lake Boone Trail
Suite 201
Raleigh, NC 27607

Nurses who specialize in substance abuse treatment.

National Nurses Society on Alcoholism
P.O. Box 7728
Indian Creek Branch
Shawnee Mission, KS 66207

CHAPTER 7

HUMAN SERVICES JOBS

VARIETY IN HUMAN SERVICES WORK

Human services is a general term sometimes used to describe the workers who serve the community health network. They try to improve the lives, welfare, and mental health of clients. Typical human services jobs are: residential counselor, case worker, social work assistant, community outreach worker, or client advocate. There are many more, spanning the whole spectrum of clients from child abuse workers, youth workers, and family support workers, to adult day-care workers and through gerontology aides. Parole officers and probation officers, as well as mental health aides, may have human services training. Moreover, once people are treated for a mental illness and are ready to return to the community, they need to be integrated into society again. (That's how the term halfway house—now more often called a group residence or residential treatment center—came into use, the idea being that people were out of the hospital and on their way back to becoming independent.) Residential counselors and managers, group activity aides, and similar job titles all fit into these settings.

A human services worker performs a wide range of tasks for a wide variety of people, including immigrants and the poor. The goal is to help clients deal more successfully with the various aspects of life that are most troublesome. First, the worker finds out what the client's needs are. Then the appropriate person, possibly a counselor or social worker, takes a client history about health, family, income, and so forth. He or she must decide if the client is eligible for benefits, using knowledge of the health care network and the social services system to make that determination. The worker may help to organize the client's finances or work with medical records. Once a course of action is decided, the worker may need to arrange for food stamps, Medicaid, or other assistance. The worker becomes a source of emotional support as well as information for the client.

Workers at community centers plan and carry out activities for groups of participants in the mental health or social services programs. They help with basic counseling or intervene in a crisis, so they must know what to advise and when to refer a serious case to a superior. They may have responsibility for a wide variety of service programs. For instance, they may provide social services such as an "open pantry" with food for the hungry and homeless or an emergency fuel program.

Human services workers carry out their assignments and receive supervision from professionals in medicine, psychology, social work, nursing education, and rehabilitation. There were 145,000 human services workers in 1990, by the government's reckoning. About 25 percent were employed by state and local governments (mainly in hospitals and mental health centers). By 1992, the government's count was up to 189,000 workers, so the field is growing. However, the growth has not been uniform. There have been ups and downs, depending on shifts in hiring practices and changes in the methods of care. In 1992 about a quarter of these jobs were in state and local governments; another quarter were in the private social services agencies; another quarter were in group homes and halfway houses supervising residents. The remainder worked in various other settings, like clinics, psychiatric hospitals, and community mental health centers.

Because of the shift in care models from traditional inpatient to outpatient and residential, it is difficult to get an accurate count of all agencies and all personnel. (See table, Where the Jobs Are, in Chapter 2.) Paraprofessional (less than a B.A.-level education) employment ebbed at times, but showed overall growth over a 20-year span. In nonhospital, multiservice, mental health organizations, there has been a steady growth from negligible numbers at the time the category began to be tracked in the 1970s to some 28,500 in 1994, according to the statistics of the National Institute for Mental Health. By way of contrast, in private psychiatric hospitals approximately 11,500 workers were counted in 1990, up from 5,600 in 1972, but down from the 1988 peak of 12,700. Perhaps the best lesson to draw from the statistics is that any job search should take into consideration a wide variety of job settings, to see what opportunities are available locally. Check state and county hospitals, private hospitals, general hospitals with psychiatric units, VA medical centers, residential treatment centers, outpatient psychiatric clinics, and mental health agencies. Many human services workers find employment in residential settings with people who need supervision around the clock (such as the mentally retarded).

Other types of job settings include group homes for the mentally ill and residential treatment centers for substance abuse patients. These drug treatment centers have become an important job source for graduates with a substance abuse specialty. They work in detoxification programs, veteran's shelters, halfway houses, outpatient clinics, hospitals, and day treatment programs. In some regions of the country, methadone clinics and alternative therapy clinics using such treatments as acupuncture have gained importance. These job settings need workers as do homes for youth orphaned by divorce, death, or family problems. Group homes may be run by public agencies or by private sector organizations.

When you are job-hunting, contact your local or state mental organizations or mental health associations. Some organizations try to keep a low profile to preserve the privacy of patients, so you may have to network with the mental health professionals in your area to find possible job openings.

The tasks of workers include interviews, observation, record keeping, counseling, and program planning. In group homes, a worker with a one-year certificate in human services and relevant experience may find work and later promotion to supervisor. A B.S. or M.S degree in human services, counseling, rehabilitation, or social work will be a valuable asset if you want to move up in the field. Community agencies use these types of workers as well. Youth counselors need assistance with administration and program planning.

While many workers have advanced degrees, there's also a need for "streetwise" workers, people who can relate to kids and troubled individuals and who've been through problems themselves and overcome them. Particularly in the areas of youth work, drug education, and rehabilitation, it may be possible for appropriate experience to compensate for the absence of an M.S. or B.S. in social work.

For example, here is a proposal recounted by Dr. Carl Bell, director of the Community Health Council on Chicago's south side. He says "the issue is how do you take kids who have been victimized by violence and turn them into good guys." He suggests parenting training. His program uses grandmothers in such a role, and he further notes that a proposal has been made to develop a program on the model of Alcoholics Anonymous to supervise youth in inner cities, with the worker jobs going to appropriately screened and trained welfare mothers. Dr. Bell, himself a former gang member who became a psychiatrist, says this is one way to improve the safety net in inner city communities, an essential part of community health care. "That's why 95 percent of the children who grow up in poverty don't become bad."[1]

In urban areas, there may be a good deal of competition for community mental health worker positions, and degreed individuals will have an advantage. You will have to examine your job search territory to find out what the opportunities and requirements are, and where your experience and talents fit in.

To advance, training is usually needed. Credentials for human services jobs are being established in a more formal way. They are also undergoing reevaluation in national projects. Ask potential employers about their requirements before committing to an educational program.

The Council for Standards in Human Service Education (CSHSE) offers program approval to human service education programs that meet the standards of the council; the National Organization for Human Service Education (NOHSE) provides educational conferences for faculty, students, and working professionals. Local chapters of the organization encourage active participation. Many state colleges and junior colleges are members, and their faculty adhere to the standards set up by these groups. An academic program that's credentialed by CSHSE and NOHSE may carry more weight with employers. Ask those in your area as part of your personal career research.

---

[1]*New York Times,* "The Experts on Different Fronts of the Battlefield Discuss Strategies," December 30, 1994.

SAMPLE MENTAL HEALTH
TECHNOLOGY CURRICULUM

Here's a typical two-year curriculum for a mental health technology worker. Students can continue after their two-year programs and work toward a bachelor's degree with colleges in their area that have cooperative agreements with the community college. In addition to the specialty courses shown, there will be varying combinations of required courses at different colleges.

Semester 1
Introduction to Psychology
Introduction to Mental Health/Human Services
Human Biology
Observation and Recording of Mental Health/Human Services
   Programs
English Composition

Semester 2
Modalities of Treatment
Mental Health/Human Services Practicum
Natural Science Elective
English Composition

Semester 3
Abnormal Psychology
Mental Health/Human Services Practicum 2
Group Dynamics
American Government and Politics

Semester 4
Seminar in Mental Health
Mental Health/Human Services Practicum 3
Sociology Elective
Intro to Creative Experience
Behavioral Management Principles and Techniques

In addition, the curriculum includes clinical practice so graduates will gain experience in supervised clinical settings.

With this kind of educational background, students go on to become residential counselors, case managers, shelter workers, job coaches, child care workers, counselors, outreach workers, skills instructors, house managers, and community support workers. Some of the employment opportunities you'd get from such a program, according to literature from the program at Northern Essex Community College in Massachusetts, include the following: mental health outpatient clinics, halfway houses, psychiatric hospitals, community residences, adolescent treatment programs, day activity programs, work activity centers, day treatment programs, day habilitation programs, early intervention programs, special education school programs, corrections, substance abuse programs, social services, shelters, vocational and rehabilitative services.

SAMPLE COMMUNITY RESIDENCE
MANAGER CURRICULUM

Another example of the training for human services workers is the community residence manager certificate program that prepares students to help people who live in group homes and have problems with activities of daily living.

Semester 1
English Composition
Introduction to Mental Health
American Government
Observation and Recording of Mental Health Programs
Group Dynamics
Mental Health Practicum 1 in Residential Services

Semester 2
English Composition 2
Introduction to Psychology
Behavior Management Principles and Techniques
Mental Health Practicum 2 in Residential Services
Elective

Employment opportunities for graduates could be found where students do their practicums—psychiatric community residences, mental retardation community residences, adolescent programs, halfway houses, homeless shelters, women's shelters, intermediate care facilities, and human service community programs.

Many recovering individuals and high-functioning people who have disabilities need work. They need the help of employment services workers. Employment services workers place applicants in suitable jobs. Some also work at community mental health centers to assist clients. In employment offices they interview potential employees, using their interpersonal skills to find out who's the best match with the job opening. At management levels they may deal with promotions and with problems of employees. Some mental health facilities for adults have multiperson departments devoted to helping the high-functioning patients obtain the kind of jobs they are capable of performing in the community. With special training in vocational rehabilitation, these human services workers can perform valuable work on behalf of the mentally ill.

SUCCESS IN HUMAN SERVICES

It is often said that careers in the mental health professions are taxing, exhausting, or prone to burnout. What is it about a job and/or a worker that leads to success and satisfaction? Of course, it's an individual matter. But a study of more than 300 social services workers was done in the late 1980s to see what the main predictors of satisfaction and commitment were.[2] One factor influencing nurses' satisfaction on the job was the technology found on the job site. Workers must be ready to use the available technology—computers, treatment methods, and so on—before they can perform well. Employee morale is high where workers are satisfied with their workplace, with the tools they have to do their jobs, and where they are committed to their employers. The study authors noted, "These results indicate that job satisfaction depends largely on the opportunity for the human service worker to use a variety of

---

[2]Charles Glisson and Mark Durick, "Satisfaction and Commitment," *Administrative Quarterly* 33, March 1988.

skills in performing job tasks and on the clarity of the requirements and responsibilities of the job."

Along these lines of thinking, you may want to focus on the organization's resources, goals, and expertise in your interviews, and ask critical questions so you find out what you need to know about the agency's work style and personnel policies. "A social worker's successful intervention in a child abuse case or successful treatment of an adolescent drug user could be as dependent on the design and administration of the organization in which the social worker is employed as on the social worker's knowledge of relevant intervention and treatment approaches," the study concluded. Be sure to ask questions about the organization, its resources, budget, and above all its success in benefiting its clients. You will want to know how effective the organization is in treating its clients and does it help them return to a normal life or help them cope better with their problems.

JOB OUTLOOK

According to the federal government's *Occupational Outlook Survey,* "Employment of human services workers is expected to grow much faster than average for all occupations through the year 2005." The reasons for this include:

- rapid turnover is continuing, especially in group homes
- number of older people is increasing
- deinstitutionalization is continuing
- public sector is maintaining average growth, mainly through replacement

Some positions will hire high school graduates, but most prefer applicants with some college preparation in human services, social work, or one of the social or behavioral sciences. Earnings are $12,000 to $20,000 a year to start; experienced workers can earn between $15,000 and $25,000 annually. Related occupations include social workers, community outreach workers, religious workers, occupational therapy assistants, physical therapy assistants and aides, psychiatric aides, and activity leaders.

FOR MORE INFORMATION

American Federation of State, County and Municipal Employees
  1625 L Street NW
  Washington, DC 20036

Council for Standards in Human Service Education
  Northern Essex Community College
  Elliot Way
  Haverhill, MA 01830

National Association for Counseling and Development
  5999 Stevenson Avenue
  Alexandria, VA 22304

National Organization for Human Services Education
  Brookdale Community College
  765 Newman Springs Road
  Lincroft, NJ 07738

The Council for Accreditation of Counseling and Related Educational Programs (CACREP) is associated with the National Association for Counseling and Development. Twice yearly it offers lists of programs in its *Directory of Accredited Programs* for those interested in M.A., Ed.D., and Ph.D. programs in counseling.

Other sources include state employment service offices; city, county, or state departments of health, mental health, mental retardation, and human resources; local community colleges with human services programs; or social services programs.

CHAPTER 8

HOSPITAL AND NURSING HOME CAREERS

Opportunities for mental health workers in hospitals are numerous and the job descriptions varied. The jobs are no longer strictly in inpatient settings. Once the hospital itself was the focus of care and the site where patients were most often treated. Now, the hospital is the hub of a health care network, and it may have clinics and services throughout a city or even a region. Several large national health care companies specialize in psychiatric services. To reduce costs, health care providers, both public and private, are opting for outpatient settings and partial hospitalization care wherever possible.

The most noticeable trend in the mental health field during the last thirty years has been deinstitutionalization, that is, releasing patients from hospitals whenever possible, and treating patients in the least restrictive way. In 1955 almost half of all psychiatric services were provided in big, institutional hospitals. By 1971, that had dropped to only 19 percent. The number of patients in state hospitals (the average daily census) dropped to below 200,000 in 1980 from 560,000 in 1955, according to statistics from the National Institutes for Mental Health.

Outpatient services have grown tremendously during the same time period. Many patients are now treated in residential settings, nursing homes, or supervised homes. Hospitals are good places to start looking for these outpatient services because they have connections to them for their inpatients who are treated and released. Moreover, despite deinstitutionalization, there are now more patients than ever, according to mental health experts. This is true in part because the population has grown since the 1950s. Thus, there's still a growing need for people who want to work in mental health careers. Hospitals offer various services. A typical psychiatric hospital in the private sector might offer the following:

school	play therapy
occupational therapy	vocational rehabilitation
substance abuse rehabilitation	electroconvulsive therapy
art therapy	biofeedback
marital therapy	psychodrama
detoxification therapy	dance therapy
music therapy	

A specialty within mental health can help you to succeed. For example, Jay Salter became a forensic psychiatric technician at Atascadero State Hospital in California. He went on to become president of the California Association of Psychiatric Technicians and today champions the role of psychiatric technicians in the profession. As he points out, most psychiatric technicians work with the developmentally disabled. They develop a different set of skills from those who work with behavioral patients who had diagnoses such as schizophrenia. Salter's facility includes patients incarcerated by the state's justice system. In return for the difficult work he did, he had the reward of seeing the successful rehabilitations of some patients and a somewhat higher pay scale in the state hospitals than in some private facilities.

PSYCHIATRIC NURSING

Some psychiatric technicians decide to enter the field of psychiatric nursing to advance their careers. The additional medical training can be valuable, especially because of the recent advances in psychiatric drug therapy. Entry-level nursing traditionally has been open to those who complete an associate degree. Work on a psych unit is not the only choice for a psychiatric specialty. An outpatient clinic is another, and a good one if the nurse plans a future in home health. Nurses' training levels determine their responsibilities and salaries.

Supervisors are likely to be nurses with master's degrees in psychiatric or mental health nursing. They work not only in hospitals but in community mental health centers, crisis intervention centers, community health agencies, nursing homes, and other workplaces. Some are in private practice. They eventually develop specialties; for example, nursing homes need nurses who can care for Alzheimer's patients who need especially close monitoring. In hospitals they are given a great deal of responsibility. In some states, they can administer medication. In a psychiatric setting, they may have to take care of patients who are confused, or irrational, even angry at the caregiver, due to the patient's mental condition.

A first step into nursing is the Licensed Practical Nurse (LPN) program, also called Licensed Vocational Nurse (LVN) in California and Texas. This designation is appropriate for careers in hospitals and home health, among other applications. It is not as advanced as a Registered Nurse (RN) program. LPNs complete a practical nursing program that lasts about a year. Because licensing is handled by state governments, requirements will differ. In California, an LVN has to pass 1,530 hours of training in a twelve to eighteen month, full-time program. Most of these programs are at community colleges. Some adult programs are offered at high schools. In fact, 20 percent of the state's approved programs are aimed at adult students. Included in the LVN curriculum of basic nursing skills is usually some course work in psychology and rehabilitation nursing. LVNs practice in psychiatric hospitals, correctional facilities, and other such settings if they want to devote their careers to psychiatric nursing. In California, nurses at state institutions can earn $13 to $16 per hour, for a salary range of $25,000 to $30,000 a year. A Texas survey of hospitals and medical centers found that nurses' median salary was $22,360 in 1992. A national survey placed median earnings at $21,900 in 1993.

A more advanced nursing career requires completion of a registered nursing program. Staff nurses working in hospitals earned more than LPNs—$16.20 an hour in private hospitals in 1991. For their additional pay and career opportunities, they had to pass a national licensing examination. Though some employers prefer B.S.N. graduates with four-year bachelor's degrees, 60 percent of registered nurses in 1991 had entered the profession with associate diplomas in nursing (A.D.N.) from community colleges, after completing two-year programs. Education for nurses gives them clinical introductions to various hospital departments, including psychiatry, so that there's an opportunity to find out what it's like to work in each department prior to graduation. The clinical experience is a vital addition to course work in medical subjects. A full-time registered nurse could expect a median annual salary of $34,424 in 1992. A national survey of nursing homes showed that nurses were earning a median $30,200 in 1993.

A nurse who wanted to go into private practice as a psychiatric specialist would need training in group therapy and individual therapy. These advanced specialists, called nurse therapists, have a great deal of independence and responsibility.

The job outlook is very good. Hospitals still report shortages of RNs. In fact, it's expected that employment of RNs will grow much faster than average for all occupations through 2005. Hospitals make up the largest sector, but most rapid growth is likely to be in hospitals' outpatient facilities and in home health care and nursing home facilities.

ACTIVITIES DIRECTOR/RECREATIONAL THERAPY ASSISTANT

Nursing homes need trained activities directors to lead activities for residents. Hospitals need recreational therapists to do the same for recovering patients in psychiatric units. Occupational and vocational rehab therapists are also in demand. Each of these professions requires assistants. The federal government's forecast is as follows: "Recreation worker jobs should also increase in the fast-growing social services industry. More recreation workers will be needed to develop and lead activity programs in senior centers, halfway houses, children's homes, and day-care programs for the mentally retarded or developmentally disabled."

In a nursing home on a typical morning, several residents may gather for a craft project with the activities director, who has planned an entire calendar full of such projects in keeping with the needs of the residents.

Elsewhere, the director of nursing, along with relatives of a resident, is involved in a care conference. Together they plan the particular care to be given to the resident. They may recommend vocational rehabilitation or physical therapy. If the resident is developmentally disabled but high functioning, he or she may do many activities. If Alzheimer's or senile dementia is involved, the resident may be restricted to a unit under careful observation and must exercise under supervision. Perhaps the resident is convalescing after a fall. A daily workout is imperative to get muscles back in working order. Other residents may have chronic illnesses with a mental component, and so the care team develops a plan together. As an activity director or a therapist, you would participate in such planning and carry out the specific instructions of the physicians.

As the senior population grows, more such therapists and the paraprofessionals who aid them will be needed in nursing homes, long-term care facilities, and hospitals. Therapy can improve the health and strength of patients and thereby boost their self-confidence. It may help them to express themselves and it is well known that exercise and activities are good ways to manage stress. (*Activities* is a broad term that encompasses crafts, music, physical recreation, drama, games, and field trips.)

Training for therapists is fairly advanced. They need a B.S. or B.A. with course work and an internship of several hundred hours. Other workers in the field include recreational group workers, who carry out the activities that therapists prescribe. In the early 1990s, there were about 32,000 recreational therapists earning an average $25,000 per year. Many states require licensure or certification. Certification is through the National Council for Therapeutic Recreation Certification.

Best Hospitals for Mental Health

McLean Hospital, Belmont, MA
Menninger Clinic, Topeka, KS
UCLA Medical Center, Los Angeles
Massachusetts General Hospital, Boston
Sheppard and Enoch Pratt Hospital, Baltimore, MD
Institute of Living, Hartford, CT
Mayo Clinic, Rochester, MN
Columbia-Presbyterian Medical Center, New York
New York Hospital–Cornell Medical Center, New York
Yale–New Haven (CT) Hospital
Source: *U.S. News & World Report.*

Mental health workers and hospital nurses at Sheppard and Enoch Pratt Hospital provide a good example of the job situation in hospitals today. Georgia Coleman is its human resources director and Carol Perlin its associate director of nursing. In the hospital, they described nurses' duties as follows—to assist with individual, family, and group therapy. Although those nurses now conduct no individual therapy, the nurses are involved in group therapy. They also do psychological education with patients and are active in treatment planning.

In planning a career, Georgia Coleman suggests that people consider mental health worker a one-level job with the outlook being for fewer jobs in hospitals but more in other settings. Her opinion is that the jobs outside the hospital, such as community mental health worker, will have more growth and "trend-power" in the future.

The minimum training for these jobs is a high school diploma, but hospitals can and do hire associate degree personnel, bachelor's degree holders, and even master's degrees for mental health workers. Many people come to get the experience of one or more years as a mental health worker. They can later use it on job applications and resumes. A next step could be into nursing.

Gradations of mental health worker careers are based on fulfillment of requirements. On-the-job training takes place during a three-month training period. Specialties include, child/adolescent; psycho/geriatric; dissociative disorders (multiple personality disorders, for example); and chemical dependency.

The workers at Pratt have a wide range of responsibilities. A majority of the job at unit level is to direct patient care, particularly in treatment planning via their input and observations about the patient. They contribute ideas about what's effective, what didn't work, and what patients are having trouble with. They organize activities of daily living, hygiene, and dressing. They assist with leisure activities for patients.

A job with more trend-power for the future, and very closely related to the mental health worker job, is community rehabilitation worker. Such workers are specialists. They do the same activities as mental health technicians, but not on a hospital unit. They are living in community housing, on and off campus. This housing—group homes, supervised living, halfway, and quarterway houses—is for the higher functioning patients. Another term for these workers is residential coun-

selor. This is a growing profession, and many students from human services programs are entering it.

"Health care will be looking for very focused skills. We'll hire social
workers, RNs, and others because staffing is going to look different; the
patients in-hospital will be sicker. The workers here will have to be
more highly skilled," said Ms. Coleman. "We see a shift from inpatient
to ambulatory care for many patients."

For nurses, education ranges from the associate degree to the master's
degree. The average starting salary for top-level nurses is $38,000 to
$40,000. On the unit, they carry out the treatment, assess case loads, par-
ticipate in planning, and do any necessary intervening. They dispense
medication, they provide psychoeducation for both the patient and family, and they participate in group psychotherapy. The number of nurses
on duty at Pratt varies by shift and unit. In addition to the nurses on duty
in the hospital, there is a nursing education instructor who trains staff.

Other nursing jobs include the nurse manager, whose task is to over-
see the nursing unit on a twenty-four-hour-a-day basis; and the shift coordinator, whose task is to coordinate nursing activities during his or her
shift.

Carol Perlin says that in the future, she sees a shift in the mode of
practice. There may be a larger demand for social workers as primary
therapists and case managers, as well as advanced practice psychiatric
nurses. They'll do more of what the M.D.s and psychologists do now.
The physicians themselves will focus on medical management and will
pay attention to the very sick patient.

Psych Aides and Nursing Aides—Jobs and Salaries in 1992.

Nursing aide jobs: 1,308,000

Psych aide jobs: 81,000

Nursing aide/psych aide full-time median salaries: $13,800 (mid 50
percent, $11,000–$17,900; top 10 percent, $23,900).

Source: U.S. Bureau of Labor Statistics, *Occupational Outlook
Handbook,* 1994–95; America's Top Medical and Human Services Jobs.

There's growth in the mental health field; however, job descriptions are changing—fewer psych aides and more nursing aides jobs are available now. Future needs will grow; job settings and job titles may change as health reform takes place in state and local mental health programs.

DOUG THOMPSON, DIRECTOR
OF HUMAN RESOURCES

Another noted hospital is Hartford's Institute of Living. Doug Thompson, director of human resources, discusses the prospects for mental health workers from his perspective.

Q. Tell me about the Institute?

A. Well, the Institute, as Hartford Mental Health Network, has five units with 140 beds. Now that includes one hospital-based unit on the main campus and four units on the former Institute of Living campus. I will tell you parenthetically that we were 420 beds and we went down to 110 beds when we merged, and added 30 back. We closed a number of our inpatient units and we reduced our staff from 1,300 to about 600 roughly, but we opened some satellite offices, one in Farmington, a residential suburban setting, and to be frank the reason we opened units outside of the city is that people are concerned about safety coming into an urban setting. And we also have east of the river an adolescent center in Enfield, CT, another suburban location, going out to where we feel the clients are located.

Q. What do you see as the prospects for a person who's just getting into the field as a mental health technician? What are the trends and what is the job outlook?

A. There are two focuses here. One, of course, is inpatient care, and for a high school graduate getting into inpatient care in psychiatry there aren't too many options. One is the mental health worker or the psychiatric aide as we now call that position. And that of course is the person who has a high school degree and whom the institution is willing to train to deliver basic care to psychiatric patients. This is the kind of care that would be given below the level of a licensed professional. Escorting patients, for example, participating in day-to-day activities with them, intervening in inappropriate behavior, providing activities of daily living, that kind of care. It does not require any college preparation. We would prefer someone with a baccalaureate in psychology, but it's not required for this mental health worker/psychiatric aide position. We will train and most facilities will train them from a week to several months, depending on the organization. At the Institute of Living we have a training course that is several weeks long that combines classroom and clinical training for those people coming in. You're teaching people how to respond to the various behaviors of someone who may be psychiatrically ill, as well as teaching them some basic nursing care—taking a temperature and reading blood pressure—which is an aspect of the job.

Q. How challenging is it physically?

A. There is some restraint when a patient is out of control. You do not need to be an Arnold Schwarzenegger. You should be able to kneel and lift easily when you're working with a patient.

Q. What goes into crisis intervention?

A. Primarily a program of de-escalation. When you are working with someone who becomes agitated, the approach should be to de-escalate the situation, rather than inflame it and cause further problems. Now part of that program is also safe-restraining techniques. We realize that not in every situation are we going to be able to talk the patient down. So it's that kind of situation where there is some practical and theoretical basis.

Q. I'd like to ask again about training. Can you describe it in more detail?

A. Right. There are several weeks of training. This is provided in our nursing education area. We have a nurse education instructor who provides the teaching, and that involves a variety of different courses on interpersonal skills training to crisis intervention training and CPR training, which is required on an annual basis.

Q. What are tasks that they are doing in a typical day? Start with psychiatric aides.

A. It would be everything from waking patients and making sure they are appropriately attired to supervising at meal times in the common dining room, to escorting patients to various activities on or off the patient unit. They would be communicating frequently with the nurses in charge. They would be communicating with the nurses regularly. They may be performing what we call one-to-one. If someone is suicidal, they would be staying with that patient exclusively on a one-to-one basis, making sure he doesn't harm himself or herself.

Q. At the other end of the spectrum, these workers are not doing counseling but some observation, so what skills are needed there?

A. Well, there is an aspect of socialization involved in terms of the level of interaction with the patient. They're therapeutically involved with the patient in terms of discussions of how they're doing, and what's going on in the here and now, and observation, but they're not doing therapy. That's all left to the professionals—a nurse therapist, a social worker, a psychiatrist or psychologist.

Q. What is the career ladder there at Hartford, if any?

A. Let me explain that prior to October 1 the psychiatric technician position was a unionized position, and within that position there were levels of psychiatric aide. Initially we had aide 1, 2, and senior, and then we collapsed it to aide and senior aide. When we merged, the titles were changed to reflect the titles that were in place at Hartford Hospital. I think you'll find throughout health care we're collapsing those career ladders and eliminating them. And you talk about trends coming, I think you'll see that more often as we have in nursing, you'll see the ladders collapsed down and eliminated particularly as censuses drop and we move to an outpatient partial model of care.

Q. How often does someone progress from psych aide to a professional position?

A. Well, it varies. It depends on what part of the country you're in. We've had a number of psych technicians who've gone on to associate nursing degree programs, and have progressed on to get their bachelor's and master's degrees in nursing. And we probably have a half a dozen on our staff who've done that in the past five or ten years. Our former vice president and chief nurse executive started at the Institute as a psychiatric aide a number of years ago and he progressed through the organization as he gained additional education. So it does happen, particularly for those folks who get into the field and find out they really like it but realize they cannot progress further without additional education. Because as I tell people who come into this job, particularly those who are in college or have college degrees, once you've been a psychiatric aide a year or two, you've learned as much as you're going to, and to progress beyond that in terms of your scope of responsibilities, you need to attain additional education and training. So it's a good job for a year or two even for someone with a college degree. And as you know, a degree in psychology will not take you very far unless you're pursuing a master's degree.

Q. Can you discuss nurses' training?

A. They can come in many different ways from education, associate degrees, or bachelor's, you have all that. They would go through a training program as well that is specific to psychiatry and would deal with how we deliver care in the Institute of Living, with regard to developing a nursing care plan; the supervisory structure, in terms of who they're working with; the types of behavior they'll be confronted with; psychopharmacology, because the medicines you'd find in a regular medical setting would be different than what you have in psychiatry.

Q. What additional responsibilities are nurses taking on?

A. The nurses are primarily working on the administration of medication, documentation, dealing with the families, and with insurance. I think nurses would back me up on this, that nurses are spending more time on documentation, because managed care companies are requiring more documentation before they will pay the bills.

Q. They need reporting skills as well as medical skills?

A. Exactly, they need to be able to document clearly. The same goes for the psychiatric aide, by the way, because they're working in a sophisticated medical psychiatric environment. And if they don't, they need to know how to find out what was said. So it is possible that an eighteen-year old high school graduate could do this job, but we would prefer someone who has had a year's experience so that they at least have the background that goes with working in a health care or acute-care setting.

Q. What are some of the possible jobs that fit that career path?

A. Well, nursing aide; you'll find that primarily in a geriatric setting, a CNA. In Connecticut at least, you are certified by the state agency. So they maintain the training at a specific level. Now the new term that's coming in, at least around here, is patient care associate. This is a more sophisticated level of hospital employee, a person who can do clerical as well as clinical functions that a nurse would not necessarily do. And what we may see is a decrease in the number of nurses in inpatient settings and an increase in the number of nonlicensed care givers. So that may create openings for people who are just coming out of school. Or, it may mean retraining for those who are currently in the system. My guess is it will be a combination of both of those.

Q. What earnings are typical in the field?

A. I would say $19,000 to a range of $25,000. Depending on whether or not unionized and the locale. And you factor in shift work and weekend differentials. So there's decent earnings potential for high school graduates.

Q. Where do you see most opportunities in mental health in the future?

A. There are several. One certainly would be the chemical dependency positions which require an associate degree with the appropriate certification as a drug or alcohol counselor. And that requires either one or two thousand hours of internship. It's a lengthy process. That's one area. And it's an outpatient-based program. It's not going to be an inpatient model. You get the patient detoxed in a few days and you get them into a partial or outpatient program. Another area is occupational therapy. There currently is a shortage in that area of psychiatry. We cannot find a therapist for love or money. Now primarily because the facilities in the disability area are paying as much as $60,000 a year for the services of an occupational therapist and because they are reimbursable [by third-party payers], it's a moneymaker—and these are bachelor's-level jobs! If I was encouraging anyone, I'd tell them to look at the chemical dependency area, to look at the occupational therapy area, and if they're administratively oriented, to look at medical records technician. Either the RRA or the ART, the registered records administrator or the accredited records technician.

Q. And this is likely to persist?

A. Yes, for the next five years at least.

Q. Is there a way the trend to community health and outpatient care would require entry-level personnel? Where are other settings where they might find employment?

A. I think mental health will be going into the home over the next five years. We'll have more of a home health aide approach. It wouldn't surprise me that if someone is depressed or if someone had a psychiatric condition that could be addressed by a home visit, we may do that, because I'm sure it would be far less costly. I know it would be. I think it will be modeled after the VNA [Visiting Nurse Association] approach. And that's already being modeled in the psychogeriatric area. As the hospitals are squeezed in terms of inpatients, they're going to become much more creative in developing this kind of program and utilizing this kind of personnel. So you may have the professional supervise the program and the paraprofessional or unlicensed person actually delivering some of the day-to-day care. And it might not be a bad business to get into right now.

Q. Can you discuss some of Hartford's outpatient programs? Are there opportunities there?

A. Yes. We do have a bachelor's-level position in Enfield. So there may be a place in these day programs for the unlicensed professional. One area I haven't touched on is residential programs. We have four of those, and these are staffed by residential counselors who are required to have a college degree.

Q. What would they major in?

A. Psychology, sociology, family relations. And these four programs are residential in nature. One is adolescent; one is professional, primarily the priest and clergy; one is for longer-term or chronic clients; and the fourth is a grant-funded program funded by the state, for patients who were in state institutions. And each program has a program manager who is a master's level professional. But the staffing is done at the bachelor's level. And they are providing counseling for the clients.

It's not as intense. It's more homelike. It's much less expensive, which is obviously more attractive to the people who pay the bills.

Q. Will health reform change the general structure of mental health care so there would be more or less need for people?

A. It depends. Originally the emphasis of reform was going to be outpatient care, with a deemphasis of inpatient care. I think that's going to continue. Over the next five years we'll see a burgeoning of the outpatient care, and there may be more opportunities for entry-level positions in the partial outpatient program. The opportunities for those will grow, just as they have on the inpatient.

FOR MORE INFORMATION

American Health Care Association
   1201 L Street NW
   Washington, DC 20005
   Information on long-term health care nursing careers.

American Nurses' Association
   600 Maryland Avenue SW
   Washington, DC 20024-2571

American Psychiatric Nurses Association
   1200 Nineteenth Street NW
   Suite 300
   Washington, DC 20036
   A resource for some information on the profession. Primarily a membership association for professional, practicing, psychiatric nurses.

National Association for Practical Nurse Education and Service Inc.
   1400 Spring Street, Suite 310
   Silver Spring, MD 20910

National Association of Private Psychiatric Hospitals
   1319 F Street NW, Suite 1000
   Washington, DC 20004

National Association of State Mental Health Program Directors
   66 Canal Center Plaza, Suite 302
   Alexandria, VA 22314

National Council for Therapeutic Recreation Certification
   49 South Main Street, Suite 5
   Spring Valley, NY 10977

National Federation of Licensed Practical Nurses, Inc.
   P. O. Box 18088
   Raleigh, NC 27619

National Therapeutic Recreation Society
   3101 Park Center Drive
   Alexandria, VA 22302

Title 38 Employment Division (054D)
   Department of Veterans Affairs
   810 Vermont Avenue NW
   Washington, DC 20420
   For government employment in Department of Veterans Affairs medical centers.

   See also Appendix B in K. Frederickson, *Opportunities in Nursing Careers,* for more information about nurses' education requirements.

CHAPTER 9

CHILDHOOD AND ADOLESCENT CARE

Only a fraction of the children and teens who could benefit from care ever enter the mental health care system. That's why there's likely to be a demand for child care workers during the next ten years. Surprisingly, no reliable national study of children and mental health has yet been done, according to the 1994 report on U.S. Mental Health by the National Institute of Mental Health, which reported that "no national epidemiological studies have been conducted in this country that would provide valid indicators of . . . the prevalence of mental disorders among children." Education experts think that from 3 percent to 5 percent of all school-age children may have some disorder, but less than 1 percent are ever identified for special education. Because the school system sees most if not all U.S. children over time, that's as close to a national assessment of the scope of the problem as exists.

What types of services to these children or teens need when they are identified, evaluated, and treated? They need services for the developmentally disabled and services for behavioral disorders. In addition to special education, several other specialized services should be available if needed, under ideal circumstances.

Assessment of developmental disabilities comes from pediatricians who work with families. Public health agencies may see such children first, if the families rely on Medicaid resources. Children with certain disabilities will need long-term care that can involve such professionals as home health aides, occupational therapists and their assistants, and nurses' aides. Mental health and substance abuse services are obviously essential for children today. If a child or teen is in serious need, treatment would take place as an inpatient in a psychiatric hospital or unit of a general hospital. For longer-term treatment of disorders or addiction, a residential setting would be ideal. If only a short-term stay is needed, partial hospitalization or day clinics may be the site of care. For emergencies, care may come from a community center, a crisis line, and/or a crisis counselor, as well as the emergency room at a hospital.

Where there are no specialized mental health agencies, other types of agencies may provide the same services, or they may refer a child in need to a specialized service for mental health care. For example, general health care providers such as hospitals or emergency rooms treat teen drug abusers with emergency medication. Public welfare agencies also often become involved in the psychosocial care giving that's needed. Finally, the juvenile justice system sometimes becomes the starting point for care. In 1992 it was estimated by one researcher that about 14 percent to 22 percent of the 848,000 juveniles in the custody of the court system needed mental health care because they had the clinical symptoms of at least one mental disorder.

Most common conditions of children with disabilities.	*Helping professions for children with disabilities.*
epilepsy	physician
cerebral palsy	psychologist
birth defects	physical therapist
mental retardation	occupational therapist
neuromuscular disease	speech pathologist
learning disabilities	public health nurse
and language disorders	school nurse
hyperactivity	pediatric nurse
	social worker

(Source: Prensky, Arthur L. and Helen Stein Palkes, *Care of the Neurologically Handicapped Child,* New York: Oxford, 1982.)

Many child workers will benefit from mental health training. Forecasts place childhood workers near the top of the list of high-growth occupations during the next decade. Government forecasts call for a sharp increase in the number of workers needed—over a million by 2005. Child care ranges from day-care workers to more specialized workers in health care institutions. A portion of these children will require specialized care.

How many children need help and what kind of help do they need? For behavioral problems, the National Institute of Mental Health estimated that for every 100,000 children there would be 10,000 who would be disturbed in some way, 200 who would be mentally ill, but only 60 would be in residential treatment centers. These are conservative estimates. It was apparent from these surveys that as many as two-thirds of the children in need of help for mental or emotional problems were not being treated. Author Richard Sauber in *The Human Services Delivery System* concluded that "these children were literally lost to the system, as they were handed from training schools to reformatories to jails and processed through all kinds of understaffed welfare agencies."

It's not clear where the money would come from to fund the needed programs. Both public and private funds will be needed. Many options have been tried. For example, a model program called the Child and Adolescent Service System Program aimed to help children and teens with severe emotional problems. The Robert Wood Johnson Foundation followed this program with a national demonstration project for youth that experimented with methods of improving care. According to Sharon Lynn Kagan in *Integrating Services for Children and Families,* programs like these may become models for future care.

If you are interested in pursuing a specialty in child and adolescent care, private psychiatric hospitals may be a good source of job possibilities because their patients are often adolescents. The federal Center for Mental Health Services found that 41 percent of the inpatient population in private psychiatric hospitals in 1988 were under eighteen. Of those in the residential treatment programs of private psychiatric hospitals, 76 percent were under eighteen. That contrasts sharply with the survey's findings in state and county mental hospitals and general hospitals, where the patient population under eighteen was much lower. Among inpatients, state and county mental hospitals counted 7 percent under eighteen, while nonfederal general hospitals had 17 percent under eighteen.

Key standards of care for adolescent care providers are:

- an individual treatment plan,
- access to educational services when treatment requires absence from regular school,

- careful planning for any transfer so that continuing care, education, and support are assessed, and
- a written policy about treatment methods.

GARY MCBRYDE, HUMAN
RESOURCES COORDINATOR

An example of a facility that treats adolescents is the Brown Schools, a unique health care and educational facility, with one of its locations in San Marcos, TX. Gary McBryde is the human resources coordinator there. This facility is widely recognized for its programs in mental health. McBryde describes the educational activities of the school as well as some recreational therapy programs.

Q. Briefly, what is the Brown Schools and what is your role there?

A. I'm the human resources coordinator at San Marcos Treatment Center, known also as the Brown Schools. Our facility has been in existence for fifty-one years. We began as a place for mentally retarded children, throughout the years evolving into a neuropsychiatric hospital that specializes in the most difficult-to-treat adolescents and young adults throughout the country.

Q. What is the range of jobs with a mental health care component?

A. At the entry level we have what we call the direct care workers, and the job classification is mental health associate; within that job classification, we at this facility have a career ladder, and generally what we look at is experience working with these types of kids, not just in the mental health field. But again, our population is the most difficult to treat.... so we look for experience...in terms of a career ladder. We have an intern level, which is a three-month period.

Q. Criteria?

A. Minimum criterion is a high school diploma. Depending on experience with this population, we train the individual to work with this type of population. Depending on experience, we have five levels, each one requiring more and more experience.

Q. Tell me some more about Brown Schools. I understand you're part of a national chain?

A. Yes. Our corporate affiliation is Healthcare America.

Q. And this is under the corporate structure, headquartered there in Austin?

A. Yes. Most of the Brown Schools part of it is in San Marcos, Austin, and San Antonio. Our program was designed as a psychiatric facility. In the corporation there are also medical-surgical hospitals, but our program, the Brown Schools, is known for psychiatric units.

Q. What is the nature of the work for the mental health technicians?

A. They work directly with our patients on a day-to-day basis. Their main job is to supervise the patients. They're primarily there to assist in the direct care and management of the adolescent and young adult patients that we have here, going by the prescribed treatment plan of the physician and the treatment team. They also, in terms of patient care, work in conjunction with the other programs designed for the total treatment of our patients, including educational programs.

Q. What are the diagnoses of the patients?

A. It could be any number of diagnoses.

Q. The workers have to be familiar with a variety of psychiatric illnesses?

A. Yes. What we get in terms of applicants are people who are in the psychology/social work field. So in terms of their initial knowledge of what types of population we have and all that, they're aware of what at least the terminology means in terms of conduct disorders. But we also provide for any new employee an initial two-week training program.

Q. Why don't you briefly describe the disorders and how you train people to deal with them?

A. Well, in terms of the training, primarily what we look at is if they've got experience with conduct disorders. I'm trying to think of the multiple diagnosis kids that we have here, of the different disorders; most of them have a primary diagnosis but there are secondary and tertiary diagnoses involved in their treatment. Again, these are not the types of kids who have just initially had problems; these are kids that have had generally a minimum of three psychiatric inpatient placements before they even get to us—and have failed at those other placements. Most of the time, it's more like nine or ten other placements or attempts in a psychiatric setting, so again we're very specialized in the population we treat. Many of our patients are involved in the sexual treatment program; we have a chemical and substance abuse program that's integrated as part of their program; we have an experiential program, a ROPES program, we provide a speech and language program.

Q. Explain what a ROPES program is?

A. It's an outdoor experiential program. "ROPES" stands for reality oriented physical experiential services. And it's a specialized form of individual and group psychotherapy. They use a series of physical initiative activities to facilitate change and growth in our patients. The course consists of ropes and cables constructed to create a challenging and unique series of different obstacles for the patients and their families; the use of it depends on what the patient and the family needs. The course challenges are built close to the ground, so a patient or a group of patients, or patients and their family have to work together to resolve how they're going to successfully complete the challenge. So it gives a lot of information about the dynamics of the family.

Q. And the speech program? Are the mental health care workers involved in each of these programs?

A. They would be involved in the support services. Each one of these programs or different modalities that I mentioned have trained people in them. Our ROPES program has people that are trained to provide those services. In the speech-language program, the person has to be master's level.

Q. Then what would be the role of the mental health workers in, for example, the drug abuse program?

A. They would provide support. If it's a group, they would be there and work with any possible behavior problems that occur. And that type of situation is more one of supervision.

Q. What about in the experiential program?

A. They may be there for supervision and to assist with whatever the therapist needs.

Q. Would we have one upper-level person and one direct-care worker?

A. The staffing pattern depends on the size of the group.

Q. What are the working conditions? What is the workweek like?

A. In terms of our daily program, our direct-care workers are shift workers: 7 to 3, 3 to 11, 11 to 7, and again depending on what their shift is, it determines what their role is. And 7 to 3, Monday through Friday, patients are in school, so they would provide supervision getting the kids to school, stay in the classroom, provide additional help for the teacher; and really that's their function during the day. We don't have a whole lot of mental health associates that work 7 to 3, Monday through Friday, primarily because our kids are supervised by our educational therapists, our teachers. From 3 to 11 they would be responsible for seeing that the kids get to their scheduled activities, whether that would be group, individual therapy, dinner, evening activities that are planned—again providing supervision during those activities. In the evening, whether it's recreational like playing basketball or going to the movies, they would be there, provide assistance and supervision of the patient.

The 11 to 7 mental health associates are designed to provide supervision and any kind of therapeutic help the patients may need. Generally 11 to 7 they do the paperwork.

Q. The paperwork? A daily report? Pharmaceuticals?

A. Right. Each mental health associate, no matter what their shift, will have some documentation to do. And that can range just from a shift report, where they give a report about how each patient did during their shift, or any other kind of documentation we have to have during that shift.

Q. To help with career advancement, what additional training should associates have?

A. Each one of the positions has minimum requirements for experience in order to move from one to the other. We have two types of training: we have our initial new employee training and orientation—that's a two-week program designed to introduce the employee to terms and concepts, the information that they're going to need. A lot of this is mandated by the various organizations that license and accredit us: Joint Commission, Texas Department of Mental Health and Retardation, Texas Department of Human Services, CHAMPUS, there are various organizations that license us. In the first few weeks they have to do forty hours of shadowing, meaning that they go to the unit with a senior member of the team and for two weeks they follow that person around. They do a lot of observations, they ask a lot of questions, they learn a lot about the processes of their particular unit and how it functions. There are classes we have designed about what they need to know: unit safety; programs they need to know, such as behavior shaping, managing aggressive behavior; all the different types of documentation they're going to have to be aware of; and first aid, CPR, and other courses.

Following their two-week orientation, each mental health associate has to complete a minimum of fifty hours of credit a year. So we provide ongoing training throughout the year. We bring in speakers; it's opened up to the whole campus. It applies toward the training hours that the Department of Human Services requires of our direct care staff.

Q. You mentioned that the upper-level workers had a mental health or social work background?

A. Most likely they're psychology majors or sociology majors. We're a college town. And the college has a social work and psychology program. They offer them both a bachelor's and a master's program at Southwest Texas State University.

Q. Could you discuss the job outlook?

A. In terms of the job outlook, I think the direct-care mental health associate type positions will be there. The market is getting extremely difficult. The third-party payers and the amount of time that kids are spending in the psychiatric setting is really decreasing, so I think one of the big changes in the market is gearing employees more toward short-term, acute-care programs. We're more of a long-term program. The stay for kids in programs has gotten shorter and shorter.

What I think you will find is more short-term, acute-care programs. And the approach is different, the training is real different because of the goals that you're trying to achieve with the patients on a lot shorter time frame. In the mental health field, and I can only speak about Texas, there are not going to be as many private facilities. Even some of the state-run facilities are being downsized. Particularly in direct care, I see a reduction in the number, because you're not going to have as many facilities.

Q. Would you discuss earnings?

A. At our entry level, for three months they would earn $4.55 an hour; after three months they would move, based on their ability to perform the job correctly, up to $5.27. Generally what you're probably looking at for a level 2 would be $6.40 to about $7.46 an hour, level 3 probably

$7.40 to $8.64 an hour, level 4 probably $8.00 to $9.00 or $9.50; and in our system a level 5 would be about $9.00 to $10.50 an hour.

Q. What's the next step up after level 5?

A. Then you start getting into your specialized areas. In our system, if they wanted to be a teacher out here they'd have to have a four-year special education certification. If they wanted to be a therapist, they would have to be a master's level social worker or a licensed practical counselor. Again, the speech department is a specialized area; you have to have the credentials. So moving to a different level is going to depend on their educational background.

Q. Let me ask about the size of your facility there. What's the average patient population and the total number of staffers?

A. We usually operate with between 225 and 250 staff. We have between 85 and 100 patients. The school is all part of our program. All of our patients are school-age or are in vocational programming here. One thing that's probably a little bit different about our program is that our teachers are employed by our facility. We do not contract with a local school district, which a lot of psychiatric facilities do.

Q. So this is a very labor-intensive operation?

A. Well, that number includes all our administrative staff. If you're just looking at direct-care staff, it would probably be 140 direct care people.

Q. Are the kids who are in school there long-term?

A. No, not necessarily. The educational program/vocational program is a service we provide while they're here. And it's a credentialed program, so they don't lose anything during the time they're here. They do get the high school credit when they go back.

MUSIC THERAPY WITH CHILDREN

Many kinds of therapy are effective in the care of this age group. Therapeutic recreation, as mentioned by McBryde, is especially useful with young people at the Brown Schools.

Another example of creative treatment is music therapy, which can be surprisingly effective. Music can sometimes draw out a response from children who previously did not respond to any other kind of stimulus. It is used in conjunction with other treatments. In *Creative Music Therapy,* by Paul Nordoff and Clive Robbins, a five-and-a-half year old named Edward entered treatment at the day-care unit for psychotic children in the School of Medicine at the University of Pennsylvania. A direct-care worker accompanied him at all sessions. He was an active child but easily upset, with many tantrums, outbursts, and panic attacks. He began music therapy as part of his treatment for psychosis and autism. At each session, a mental health child care worker would sit with him and hold or even carry him when he wished, as the therapist played piano or tried a variety of musical instruments with the child. At first, the therapist tried to take Edward's movements or sounds and accompany it with music to gain contact. Edward began to sing along with the music at the third session. The therapist made up participation songs for him. Edward was less fearful, although he still had tantrums. Later, he began singing along with a "hello song" and stayed attentive throughout the session. (His mental I.Q. was equal to age three.) After nine sessions he repeated the names of objects after his child care worker prompted him. After seven months, (with music therapy and other therapy) he used 120 words including verbs and short phrases. By age nine, he was ready to be discharged from the day-care unit and enrolled in a special school.

Under the current system, the responsibility for child and teen mental health may divided among several public and private agencies. A job search for an entry-level job has to cover as many of these as fit the worker's background, skills, and interests. In addition to facilities like Brown Schools, examples of agencies that treat children with mental disorders or care for them are hospitals, schools, foster homes, residential treatment centers, substance abuse or chemical dependence clinics, and detention centers in the juvenile justice system.

Many entry-level workers will be needed to help children and teens through the healing process required to overcome mental illness or to live with disabilities in their many forms. Until more is known about the extent of the needs and the best methods of treatment, it is difficult to say specifically what kind of training will be most valuable. Training as a mental health technician is one option. Advancement in a school setting will require special education training. Substance abuse treatment is now a recognized specialty, and counselors can receive certification. Child welfare agencies will need human services workers and others.

FOR MORE INFORMATION

American Art Therapy Association, Inc.
  1202 Allanson Road
  Mundelein, IL 60060

American Association for Music Therapy
  P.O. Box 80012
  Valley Forge, PA 19484

American Dance Therapy Association
  2000 Century Plaza, Suite 108
  Columbia, MD 21004

American Occupational Therapy Association
  P.O. Box 1725
  1383 Piccard Drive
  Rockville, MD 20849-1725

Child Care Employee Project
  6536 Telegraph Avenue, A201
  Oakland, CA 94618

Children's Home & Aid Society

  A public/private, long-lasting program from foster care to institutionalized care. Check local offices in various cities.

Council for Exceptional Children
  1920 Association Drive
  Reston, VA 22091

  Write for a list of training programs in special education.

Federation of Families of Children's Mental Health
  1021 Prince Street
  Alexandria, VA 22314-2971

National Association for the Education of Young Children
  1509 Sixteenth Street NW
  Washington, DC 20036

National Association for Music Therapy
  (NAMT)
  8455 Colesville Road, Suite 930
  Silver Spring, MD 20190

National Association for Retarded Citizens
  2709 Avenue E East
  P.O. Box 6109
  Arlington, TX 76011

CHAPTER 10

DEVELOPMENTAL DISABILITIES IN ADULTS

BARBARA FRANK, PERSONNEL MANAGER

Care for adults with developmental disabilities has an innovative spirit at The Lambs, Inc., a national center for people with mental retardation. The 120 residents of their rural/suburban setting in northern Illinois are moderately to mildly mentally disabled. Some work at The Lambs Farm restaurant and shops, a commercial complex built near the residences. Others work in the surrounding communities. After their day's work, they return to group homes or a dorm at The Lambs. It takes a staff of about 180 people to work at the homes, restaurant, and shops. Entry-level jobs include direct care, residential workers, and daily living aides; upper-level jobs, such as residential manager in a group home, are also available at a facility such as this one. "Habilitation" aides are those who help residents develop their skills to their fullest potential. Barbara Frank, personnel manager, answered the following questions.

Q. What age group are your residents?

A. They have to be at least eighteen.

Q. So they're through with school?

A. No. In Illinois, persons with mental disabilities may remain in school until they are twenty-two years of age.

Q. For direct care, the basic mental health worker position, what would be the requirements?

A. It's an entry-level position, there aren't any specifics as far as training goes. We like to have somebody who's had some background working with the mentally retarded.

Q. What special training would be needed in general for workers here?

A. It's on-the-job training, plus we require a habilitation certificate. They must hold a current Illinois habilitation aide certificate or the equivalent.

Q. Where would they get that certificate training?

A. Lambs has a certified training program. Also, it's available at a two-year college with an accredited program.

Q. What do you look for, what are the skills that the direct-care people have that make them good and effective workers?

A. On the job, the main thing is to be able to deal with the participants, act appropriately in a stressful situation, and to follow the active treatment programs for the participants which are designed by the professional staff with input from the direct-care staff. That's pretty much the on-the-job training.

Q. Who are the other members of the care team?

A. It is called the interdisciplinary team, which consists of the habilitation specialist, the habilitation supervisor, direct care, therapeutic assistant, case manager, and others.

Q. Is there a career ladder that would lead from direct care to a specialist position?

A. You need a degree. Yes, you could start out as direct care, but then you'd have to be working toward your degree. We do have a young lady right now who's been a direct care for four years, and she's going to school right now for her degree. We made an exception in her case because her experience far outweighs anybody coming in with a degree.

Q. What you look for, ideally?

A. Human services.

Q. What types of clients are they working with?

A. These are the participants who are higher functioning and live in the homes here. A daily living aide and direct care overlap in what they do. The daily living aide does a lot of transporting of participants to doctors' offices for appointments and communicating with the doctor or the nurse to find out what the diagnosis is and about what needs to be done and bringing that information back to the nurse (at The Lambs Farm) and all the paperwork that goes with that. They transport them to anyplace that they happen to be going, if they're going on vacation or to the train. It's a lot of one-on-one contact because they're in the car alone with them, but the only requirement we have is a valid driver's license, violation-free for the past twelve months.

Q. What's a day like for a direct-care worker?

A. The first shift starts at about a quarter to seven in the dorm and continues until three. And the job is to make sure the participants are up and that they take care of their morning routines. They go over to the restaurant for breakfast, so it's walking over there and supervising, making sure they're there and they eat and they get their lunches, and go to their jobs around the farm. So it's a supervisory job. If there are any participants who are not able to work, the direct-care person monitors them at the dorm.

The afternoon person is responsible for leisure activities; they play games. The participants do clean their own rooms, but they need the supervision of someone to help them, so that's what the direct-care person does.

Q. Describe the therapeutic assistant's day?

A. The therapist is not a staff position, it's a consultant position. The assistant here is following the direct written procedure of the therapist. It's structured for them, when during the day and what they're going to be doing with them.

Q. Anything else you could mention about the daily living workers? They deal with transportation and activities?

A. ...A couple of them come in at seven in the morning and they work from seven to nine A.M. in the group home. And that's making sure the participants are up and that they're making their lunches and getting their breakfasts, that they're dressed properly, and going out to work. They're dealing with twelve adult participants each.

Q. These two workers are part-time or full-time?

A. They are full-time. They work two hours in the group home, and from nine until three is when they do their daily living work and transporting.

Q. Who are the other workers in the group homes?

A. We also have house managers. Ideally we'd like to have college graduates, whose degree is in the social services area. Those positions can be live-in or not. It depends on their needs. All the homes have apartments where the live-in staff can live. House managers work in the evenings from two to ten or four to ten if they're live-in, and the live-in house managers have the seven to nine A.M. shift. Their responsibility is monitoring training in areas of food preparation, making sure participants do their assigned duties, such as cleaning their rooms. It's taking them for their weekly outings. They go out into the community at least once a week for dinner or shopping. It's helping them balance their checkbooks.

Q. What would the range of pay be for these workers?

A. Direct care I believe is $7 hour; daily living aide, $6.50; house manager is $8 to $8.50.

Q. Do you have social workers on staff?

A. Those are all college-degreed positions. Our case managers have to have at least one year's clinical experience with this population—adults with mental disabilities or the developmentally disabled.

Q. What is your main funding source? Based on your experience, what would you say the future of this field is? Will there be some changes because of possible health reform?

A. Our main source is through donations. Obviously we get some help through the federal and state government. It's really difficult. We have a few corporate sponsors. We have a log of fund-raisers. There are so many good organizations, good groups that need money, it's become much more difficult to get the donations, so it's an ongoing concern. I don't know how there'd be fewer jobs in the field in the future. There are so many people who need care. The problem with this field is that it is very low-paying. A lot of the turnover is caused by burnout. It's a big problem. You can really see it in the dorm. A lot of the people can only deal with it for so long. We see it in direct care.

Q. Is there any way the profession has found to combat that?

A. I'm sure there are programs out there. It takes a special person to work in these types of facilities, one who is extremely caring, nurturing, and isn't out to make a whole load of money. And we have had longtime staff, because they do become like family. It is their home.

Q. Are there any changes in the mental health field that we should be aware of? new ideas? new treatments?

A. The main thing that a place like Lambs is trying to do is put these people on a competitive plane. Go around to the stores and you'll see disabled people working. Years ago they were hidden in the back room or thought to be stupid and they couldn't do anything. So the end goal is to put them out on a competitive plane, and that's not going to change. I see this field growing, I don't know how it cannot. So many people are going to need help. Years ago families used to take care of their children, but it's becoming much more difficult.

Q. Why? Is it because there are so many two-earner families with less time for direct care?

A. Not always. The current goal is to have adults with mental disabilities live at home until they are finished with school (age twenty-two in Illinois) and then have them live in a small group home setting (four to eight individuals).

Q. Are there some success stories, in terms of going out and getting a job?

A. We have quite a few of them. We have people at Marshall Fields, one who used to work at Fort Sheridan; they work at Allstate. We have a three-person department who all go out and go to different companies, to sell Lambs and to sell the participants, and then we take the participants out there and train them.

Q. Now your latest venture is a home for the aged?

A. It's something we desperately need. We have participants that have been with us twenty-five to thirty years. We're not set up to take care of the aging population. Part of our criteria is that participants must work. Well, after they get to sixty-five they won't work, they won't want to work. And they need some additional care, so that's why we started looking into this. It's not only the facility but all the programs that go along with it that are going to be geared to a geriatric operation. We have six or seven or our own participants who will probably move into the facility. Two just left recently because they were of the age where they couldn't work anymore, and we didn't have the right programs for them.

JANET PRINDLE, ASSISTANT ADMINISTRATOR

A different experience of adult mental health care is that of a community health organization that treats behavioral problems and serves an entire community or "cachement area" as part of the public health sector's social safety net. The following interview is with Janet Prindle, M.S.W., assistant administrator of the Adult and Child Guidance Center of St. Francis Hospital in Evanston, Illinois.

Q. What's it like working at a hospital-based community mental health facility like this? What type of training do you have?

A. What's different today than when I graduated is the use of bachelor's-level social workers to do case management as opposed to therapy. Somebody needs to be available to hook clients (patients) up with other kinds of services that are lacking—either helping them get paid social security or health care—and bachelor's-level people are used for that function. The other reason that there seems to be more of a need for case management is that the mentally ill population used to stay in the hospital much longer. Now they're being released much sooner and are needing support services besides medication and counseling.

Q. About this center, and generalizing if you want to, we want to know what careers will be available five to ten years from now. What's the mission of this center?

A. Our mission is to serve the indigent and those in need of psychiatric services. We offer services for the individual, families, couples, groups, and medication services; we serve people with mild emotional disturbances and with major character disorders. We provide mental health services to people in need.

Q. How is the center funded and administered?

A. It's publicly funded by the state department of mental health. We contract with them to serve a certain number of patients. We're also funded by the city of Evanston, and also because we're running a hospice, supported by the hospital, as well.

Q. In a situation like this, what kind of a team do you put together?

A. Most of our staff are master's-level social workers, the minimum degree to do psychotherapy [author's note: with a license, as required in Illinois]. Entry-level staff need a master's in social work. We have a couple of B.S.W.s to work as case managers; they would not do psychotherapy. We have two psychologists, three psychiatrists. The social workers and the psychologists perform the same duties. They do phone intake, see people for treatment, and do the referrals. When someone is not appropriate here, we do provide them with information about other community agencies, crisis intervention, and even some case management. The only difference is that our psychologists do psychological testing. They will see couples, families, groups. I think that's unique to our center. In some agencies the responsibilities—there's more of a hierarchy.

Q. There's a sharing of responsibilities here?

A. Yes. In terms of career ladders here, the ladder starts with the basic-level social worker, then there's the clinical or administrative coordinator, where I am. And for psychologist, there isn't psychologist one, two, three; just psychologist. In terms of a typical day here, clinicians are responsible on a rotating basis to do phone intake and if someone's not eligible here to provide referrals to agencies in the person's cachement area. To do treatment planning, diagnostic assessments, crisis intervention, ongoing treatment, each therapist spends at least an hour with a supervisor on clinical and administrative issues, and also spends an hour a week with a psychiatrist about those patients who are on psychotropic medications.

Q. That's becoming more important, isn't it?

A. Yes it is. The other area that's being utilized more is partial hospitalization programs: for people who are in a crisis, at risk of being hospitalized, but cannot be maintained outside a hospital without individual support. So it's in the middle, between having outpatient and inpatient treatment, there's partial hospitalization. It's an intensive three- to five-day program where people are seen individually or in groups—we have this partial hospitalization. So those people are getting more attention and . . . it's less expensive to maintain.

Q. Can you tell me how this agency interacts with other agencies to provide services?

A. We certainly have a strong tie to schools in the area. To the homeless; some churches in the area refer homeless to us. We're close to the community, other agencies feel very comfortable referring people to us.

Q. What is the homeless care situation here?

A. We have a case manager who works with the homeless in the hospitality centers. Our cachement area is Evanston, but some of the Chicago homeless population think that if they come to Evanston they'll get better service, so that's become an issue.

Q. What is the definition of mental health/mental illness? Who gets treatment?

A. Our definition is rather broad. We would not refer to someone who's stressed out and indigent as mentally ill. We generally think of someone who is mentally ill as someone who's just been hospitalized, or is not in touch with reality. But we would serve the worried well. It's really anyone who feels out of sorts or needs to come a few times to work out a problem in their lives. It's short-term, maybe crisis intervention for some people. For other people it's long-term.

Q. Could you discuss training and skills?

A. When we hire someone we make sure they have an M.S.W. There needs to be an openness to other persons. We want to know, when they come here right out of school, are they willing to learn? There needs to be a balance between the academics and who they are as a person. Are they someone who's going to respond readily to the needs of the clients' personalities?

Q. What are the typical earnings?

A. The NASW (National Association of Social Workers) has their own standards, which are higher than the reality, but I think for the M.S.W. the starting salary should be around $25,000; here at the guidance center it's around $25,000, but at a community mental health center it's closer to $22,000.

Q. If someone's in an associate degree program, you'd advise them to go on with more education—a B.A. or an M.S. in psychology?

A. Most definitely. In order to practice here, you have to have at least an M.S.W. and be working on getting your first license, which is an L.S.W., and after supervision your L.C.S.W., and after that there's a new credential and that's getting to be a diplomat in social work. So the trend is to become more credentialed and to use people who have credentials.

Many opportunities for mental health care workers are available in facilities like The Lambs and the Adult Guidance Center. These are examples of how mental health care takes place in very different settings. Making adult mental health care a focus of your career plans, you may find that working with people who are developmentally disabled is the most rewarding to you. Or you may prefer an agency where you are close to a community, serving a wide-ranging variety of cases.

FOR MORE INFORMATION

American Mental Health Fund
  Woodburn Medical Park
  Suite 335
  3299 Woodburn Road
  Annandale, VA 22003-1275

Mental Illness Foundation
  7 Penn Plaza
  New York, NY 10001

National Alliance for the Mentally Ill
      (NAMI)
  2101 Wilson Boulevard
  Suite 302
  Arlington, VA 22201

National Alliance for Research on
      Schizophrenia and Depression
      (NARSAD)
  60 Cutter Mill Road
  Suite 200
  Great Neck, NY 11021

National Association of Social
      Workers
  750 First Street NE
  Suite 700
  Washington, DC 20002-4241

National Mental Health Association
  1021 Prince Street
  Alexandria, VA 22314-2971

CHAPTER 11

PUBLIC HEALTH AND PRIVATE SECTOR CHOICES

Another way of looking at the health care field is either through the public health care approach or the private sector health care approach. A significant career decision is whether to work with a public sector or private sector agency. Public health agencies fulfill a mission to help the neediest, regardless of their ability to pay. A career track progresses through public sector jobs via seniority, so your decision can affect your opportunities for advancement. Pay scales are based on state or federal salary schedules.

Likewise, the private sector offers a choice: some care providers are nonprofit, aiming to serve a wide public; some, especially those with a religious affiliation, strive to serve the poor. Others serve a private clientele on a for-profit basis and attempt to give the highest-quality care, which is often high-cost care, on a fee-for-service basis, or on a contract basis. Managed mental health care handled by private companies on a contract basis is an expanding field. Employee Assistance Plans (EAPs) are becoming an essential part of the employees benefits that workers for corporations expect. All of these providers need staff, and it is worth some reflection to decide where your talents and career goals are leading you: the public sector or the private sector.

PUBLIC SECTOR MENTAL HEALTH SERVICES

Because the mental health of citizens is a public policy, a large number of services are carried out by the government. It's estimated that about 15 percent of adults and 12 percent of children will experience a psychiatric disorder in any given month. Many may not have their own health insurance, and so they must turn to public hospitals and social services for help. Many mental health care services are provided at the county level, especially in areas where there's no big city with regional health centers. Let's discuss that with Karen Lake, a county mental health director in Illinois.

KAREN LAKE, COUNTY MENTAL HEALTH DIRECTOR

Q. Describe your county's mental health department?

A. We're a community health agency and primarily provide outpatient services. We do have some inpatient services in our substance abuse side of things, and we have a respite program, which is an overnight type of program that's in between hospitalization, and we have some residential type programs. But most of our entry-level positions would be at the bachelor's degree level—related to human service issues in social work or in psychology.

Q. Anything below that which would be a foot in the door?

A. I know we do hire below a bachelor's level in our residential program; those usually require some experience or an associate's degree. A residential worker is there at all times to provide coverage. That's not to negate their importance in working with the clients or their interaction with the clients, but they would not be as involved in making decisions regarding treatment, that kind of thing. . . .

Q. Could you tell me about the residential program? the people and the facilities?

A. We have a group home which works with adults who have a serious mental illness. These people stay in our group home facility and they generally are involved in some kind of programming or work or school activity during the daytime. The goal is that they will develop enough independent living skills that they could be able to transition into an apartment in the community with supervision on a daily basis.

Q. When you say "a serious mental illness," what is the range of diagnoses involved? Is that a primary diagnosis? What is the range of problems involved?

A. Schizophrenia, manic depressive, severe personality disorders, borderline personality disorders, schizo-affective disorders.

Q. Is this home open to anyone in the county?

A. Anyone who is eligible based on their mental health needs and if it looks like the programming would meet their needs.

Q. Who are the people who run the homes?

A. There's a group home coordinator and he has a master's degree. There are group home counselors, I think most have bachelor's degrees. Then there are the workers that help provide the coverage, the equivalent of a mental health technician, they could have less than a B.A. degree; if they have less, then generally four years of experience are required.

Q. Is there a training program?

A. There's more like an on-the-job training; it's not a formalized "you take this step and then that step." But we use a variety of methods. In terms of the supervisor, we have written materials, co-workers in the team (who provide answers to new workers' questions), videotapes, and those kinds of things.

Q. Is there a network for these positions at entry level?

A. We've had several people who worked here as summer interns . . . and if they're good, they'd have a shot at that job.

Q. What is your mission as a public mental health service? What makes you different, as opposed to a private hospital?

A. Basically to provide assistance to the mentally ill, regardless of their ability to pay for services. I would insert the words "provide assistance and services in a quality manner." We do keep a high standard of quality. We have very rigorous standards we have to comply with just to get funding sources. Even though we do get money from the state, or from Medicaid services that we provide, their standards are quite rigorous. We try to provide high-quality services and a very wide range of services, too. Some of the private agencies may not be able to provide the wide range that we are able to do. Case management, day programs, traditional outpatient therapy, psychiatric medication monitoring, twenty-four-hour emergency counseling. We can provide all those things plus some of the residential programs. We have a medical detox and rehabilitation programs for people with substance abuse problems and an outpatient substance abuse program, a longer-term program for women with substance abuse problems. Women can actually bring their kids to stay with them so that the mom gets treatment and the kids get treatment, just by virtue of the fact that they were having problems and they were being brought up in an environment where substance abuse was an issue. We have moms come in for treatment who might not have been able to if they had to try to find alternative care for the children. And we've got case management programs for women in the childbearing years, have young kids, or are pregnant, and have substance abuse problems.

Q. You offer a wide range of services. How much help is available in the county? Is the mental health network private as well as public? Is the system stretched to its limits?

A. There are some private providers in the community and some non-profit private providers that provide services on a sliding scale or receive money to enable people with limited income to receive services.

It's necessary for public officials to coordinate their efforts at mental health care. Interagency cooperation is a priority because people want government to serve the public with less bureaucracy. At the city level, there are often local mental health services that represent the state's effort to provide the help that is needed.

For example in Los Angeles in the 1970s, a plan for mental health services was developed by the county department of mental health to deal with the various communities within the vast urban area. Beginning with a complete community analysis, the mental health department was to implement a program that would asses the community's effect on its people. In cooperation with community groups, the department was to find ways to reduce the factors that led to stress and alienation. Educational efforts were planned to promote mental health awareness. The department wanted to let people know about social services offered by the city that could help them before they reached a crisis point. Emergency services were also to be developed in accordance with the state of the art crisis intervention. Rehabilitation services would serve patients who were recovering from a crisis. That in brief was the outline of the mental health plan. (For more information about it, see Richard Sauber's book, *The Human Services Delivery System.*)

The public sector's job is to attempt to build a system that will deal with mental illness in the general population and contribute to the development of conditions right for mental health in the community. As history has shown, in the 1990s much remains to be done, and some, though outside the scope of mental health department activities, is essential to its success. In L.A., the coordination of efforts was made with other agencies whose job it was to control gangs like the Bloods and Crips, to eliminate the illegal drug trade, and to alleviate poverty in Los Angeles, all elements that contribute to the caseload of the mental health department—an awesome task. The recognition of this agency interdependence led to efforts for reform in the state's mental health programs, coordinated at the state level. Although health reform had not yet been accomplished by the federal government, California began planning its own reforms based on a managed care model, with the mental health component included.

MANAGED MENTAL HEALTH CARE

Medi-Cal

Managed mental health care is becoming the preferred system of care nationwide. Managed care tries to reduce costs to a minimum, while not sacrificing quality or access to care. California is a prime example of the managed care model as applied to a state Medicaid program. The state has designed a new system that emphasizes continuous primary care rather than episodic crisis care of the mentally ill.

Under the enabling legislation, the Medi-Cal mental health program was totally remodeled. The state set out to build a new system that would "improve beneficiaries' access to quality services while acting as a prudent purchaser of services." Each county in the state had the choice to set up its own plan or to contract with a provider of mental health services to provide coverage.

Beginning in 1993, phase one of the plan expanded services, reorganized finances, and focused on improving quality. Phase two, in 1994, consolidated state funding of mental health services at the county level. Phase three was set to begin in 1997, when it was expected that managed care contracts would be in place throughout the state.

Some of the services the state would fund were: acute psychiatric inpatient services, long-term care, and services of psychiatrists and psychologists. The state's department of mental health was to work as a partner with various state and federal agencies on issues of financing and quality care. A statewide steering committee advises the department.

The Medi-Cal mental health plan is one of the largest programs of its kind since California has become the most populous state in the Union. In 1991 to 1992, for example, 7,500 people were in state hospitals and 320,000 people were clients in community mental health programs. The Department of Mental Health budget was more than $1.2 billion. Of this total, most went to community mental health programs, with $225 million directed to hospital programs. The state hospital system must house both the severely ill, referred by the community mental health centers throughout the state, and the criminal mentally ill population (also called the forensic population). The Department of Mental Health operates four state hospitals and provides mental health services at other hospitals through interagency agreements. About half of patients are referred through civil commitment procedures, and the other half is the forensic population.

Every state has to develop a program to provide mental health services. At the state level in Illinois, as another example, the state also faces a large task with a major urban population and a wide rural area to serve, not only with state offices but with links to community mental health organizations. The budget for 1991 included $330 million in annual grants to 380 community agencies.

In Illinois, reform measures were made primarily to make the system more responsive and to eliminate red tape. State-level commissions deal with all aspects of mental health. The ongoing effort in Illinois is to make these groups work together better, while allocating scarce funds as fairly as possible.

There's plenty of room for improvement. The Chicago Department of Children and Family Service has been criticized for problems in handling social services to children of the poor. Pressure is on the state and local agencies to provide quality service with limited funding.

In the 1970s and 1980s, many states tried to coordinate the various kinds of mental health, social welfare, and education programs through state departments of mental health. For example, Illinois created an interagency task force to tackle alcoholism and other drug dependency.

Future Trends

Federal-level welfare reform could toughen up requirements for aid of various kinds. The "welfare safety net" may not be spread as wide as before. Job hunters should keep attuned to the legislation that affects public sector funding of mental health-related agencies. Many people like the kind of helping work that public agencies do, but they have to be prepared for budget battles and public debates over their agencies' performance.

PRIVATE SERVICES

At the other end of the spectrum of health care services are the private psychiatric hospitals that seek to provide highest-quality care to patients with mental diagnoses. Most of the growth in the total number of mental health organizations in the United States from 1970 to 1990 came in the private sector. Included in this total of more than 5,000 organizations are 466 private psychiatric hospitals (as of January 1990). A survey of the patients in these hospitals showed that at year-end 1990, about 30,000 persons were receiving inpatient care. Residential treatment of private hospitals totaled 2,615 patients, while partial-care programs were caring for about 10,000 patients. Outpatient programs handled about 85,000 cases. That's a snapshot of the system. During the whole year, the nation's private hospitals reported 431,473 inpatient care episodes.

According to this survey, conducted by David Brown Associates for the U.S. Mental Health Yearbook in 1994, the most frequently encountered services in a private psychiatric hospital are child, adolescent, adult, older adult, and alcohol/drug abuse programs. The hospitals offer individual, family, group, and recreational therapies. These programs are very labor intensive. Full-time staff numbered almost 65,500. There were more than 12,500 nurses (RNs) and 25,000 other mental health workers.

Because private hospitals offer a wide range of services, from schools to residential care, they will need staff in a variety of positions, from psychiatric technicians to vocational rehabilitation aides, from nurses to group home managers. Admission of more Medicare and Medicaid patients to private hospitals is one trend that could affect the type of staff needed. In recent years, these government program patients comprised nearly 40 percent of all patients. They are often older and sicker and will require longer stays in the hospital.

A private hospital can provide services the state or county can't afford. In combination with a research program, it can extend the frontiers of psychiatric medicine.

DR. WILLIAM A. SCHEFTNER, MEDICAL DIRECTOR

A new program that is attempting to bring together academic researchers and clinicians—those mental health specialists who treat patients—is the Rush Institute for Mental Well Being in Chicago, where Dr. William A. Scheftner is Medical Director.

Q. How did you get into the field?

A. My medical degree was from the University of Wisconsin, and I then had a surgical internship, then followed two years in the army, in Vietnam. I then got out, worked a year, took a residency, and came to Rush in 1976.

Q. I gather that you have a special focus in establishing the Institute?

A. To my mind we do. I think we're attempting to provide a gathering place if you will for people who can treat virtually every aspect of psychiatric disorder. I think it's no secret that a substantial portion of that is related to biological intervention, such as psychopharmacology; but there is substantial interest in the psychotherapeutic process as well. We have several projects that are attempts to investigate the process of psychotherapy. My interests tend to be affective disorders, depression, mania.

Q. What would you say to people entering the field now at the B.A. or less than B.A. level?

A. First of all, given the thrust of psychiatry, in the sense that it's being shaped and directed by managed care, you're going to find a lot more utility and more emphasis on the use of people like RNs using the old-fashioned, the old visiting nurse model that's been renamed and somewhat glorified now. It's called Home Health, but I think you'll find that nurses have already been placed in positions of substantially more responsibility because they're going out and semi-independently evaluating patients vis à vis their current functioning and status, side effects of medication—just a host of things that in the past were exclusively done by MDs and were done primarily in the hospitals. I think it's driven economically. You have to remember, the whole thrust of managed mental care is to do more with less. And to switch as much functioning as possible to lower-paid professionals. Nurses, I think, have already been put in a much tougher position.

Q. Let's talk about the Institute, and the need for it in Chicago?

A. I think that the niche in Chicago is that there is not an institution in which treatment and research have an interchange and a mutual enhancement that permits some growth on both parts. There are places that do research, but the interaction with clinicians is fairly minimal. The important thing here is there's a flow of information back and forth from things that come out of the research down to the clinical field and vice versa. For instance, the use of naltrexone in the treatment of alcoholism, the use of selective seratonin uptake blockers for disorders such as obsessive compulsive disorder, and they're sometimes found to be helpful in children with autism or adults with autism. So the point is there has to be that back and forth flow, and that's a pretty rare commodity.

Q. In terms of staffing, what will the Institute be like?

A. For staffing, we'll have an evaluation or consultation service that's going to allow us fresh looks at patients that other practitioners in the city refer for consultation. We will have the capacity for unusual forms of therapy. The staffing is going to be predominantly psychiatrists and psychologists, there will be and are social workers and substantial numbers of nurses, particularly in the investigation of new, unique antidepressants, antianxiety agents, and so on.

Q. What will happen to the technician-level jobs, now that there are fewer inpatient psychiatric units?

A. I think those individuals will be shifted to outpatient functions. They will be involved in day hospitals, in community outreach programs, in which, for instance, the highest paid individual will do the assessment, the treatment program, and the mental health worker will, for instance, carry out 50 or 60 percent of the program.

Q. Supervising activities?

A. A good example is an individual with a bad phobia. Many times they're afraid to leave the house. What you do is try to develop a series of graded exercises, and it doesn't take an RN to meet them at the next bus stop, or to accompany them on a shopping trip or what have you. There's going to be a need, but the setting will change.

Q. What do you see ahead for the field? Health reform or reform in managed care?

A. I think it's being done regardless at the state level. A number of states have their public aid patients enrolled mandatorily in HMOs and in other organizations which use pretty obvious managed mental health techniques.

The private sector is adopting the principles of managed care for all aspects of health care—employee benefits and mental health, too. Managed care methods keep costs under control for employers and providers.

DAN COHEN, REGIONAL MANAGER
OF CORPORATE OPERATIONS

The field of managed mental health care services is an expanding one. Here, Dan Cohen talks about his experience. He began as a psychiatric aide in a hospital and moved through various jobs until he became associated with managed mental health care companies that were beginning to grow around Chicago. He is now regional manager of corporate operations for Creative Care Management and a certified employment assistance professional.

Q. How do you define managed mental health care?

A. Managed mental health care. I would define it as a way of insuring cost-effective mental health treatment and also the best possible way for the client or the patient to get the best services in a cost-effective way.

Q. How is that a change from the past?

A. In the past—and I'm going back as far as the sixties—back in the 1960s and 1970s when people had emotional problems or mental health problems, they used to be institutionalized. And I'm talking about specifically the chronic mentally ill. They were institutionalized and put in state hospitals forever. And either their insurance or the state or federal government paid for them forever and ever. And due to that, and deinstitutionalization to some extent, then those people went out into the communities, [because] there were cutbacks, because there was no money for those people to stay in those services. Then, each individual community mental health center and the insurance companies decided that we needed to start looking at a way of servicing these people. It is a trend and a feeling that the cost went up because the system was being abused, and we started cutbacks. We said wait a minute we can't pay everything, it's not something that's necessary, it's not clinically or medically necessary for someone to stay in the hospital for eighteen months just to contain them. And we have research that just because a person is ill and needs some psychiatric treatment, they don't need to be institutionalized or in the hospital to be treated. They can effectively be treated on a short-term basis to be stabilized and then put them back into their community or into their own environment. Because we realize the environment has a lot to do with it. At the same time, there is a lot of relearning and retraining. If we retrain the person in the hospital, isolated, and then we send them right back into the environment where they were, there's no way of really helping them because they go back to that same sick environment. So we have been doing this in managed care. We try to get people out of the hospitals, the inpatient treatment, so they can learn how to function in their environment, in their homes, in their family, in their lifestyle.

Q. What alternates have been created to replace institutionalization?

A. I believe we have used the term partial hospitalization or day hospital. In essence it is the same type of services—the therapy, the interaction, the learning behavior, the changing behavior, the monitoring; however, the patient will be at the facility during the day, and at the end of the day the patient will go back to their home and interact with their own people, their own family. The other side of that is if something gets triggered back home, the next day we can process that and work on it, or we can say how about if we try this approach. It's a constant process, it's a relearning. Also we have intensive outpatient, and it could be that the person would be seen—instead of being in the hospital for five days or ten days—they will be seen by a therapist on a daily basis for a week or so or three times a week, and it may be more like one to two or three hours a day, and depending upon their issue. That is another modality. There is a residential facility. I am focusing on mental health, however, we have the same thing on substance abuse. In the old days, you used to go into a hospital to be detoxed, or a treatment center for a detox for twenty to thirty days. Now that person will be detoxed in one to five days to get the chemicals out of their system, monitored medically, then discharged and immediately we get them into an environment to learn coping skills to deal with the illness, the disease, and not just have a Band-Aid and say "go out and do it on your own;" there they have that support on a daily or weekly basis. And then there is after-care, too.

Q. What jobs will be important in this model of mental health care? What does this mean for the jobs in the mental health field? What are the core disciplines and what will happen to entry-level positions?

A. For the entry level it definitely will be someone with experience and a bachelor's degree in psychology, social work, or human services or a related field; nurses with experience in psychiatric services, occupational therapists, recreational therapists, social workers, psychologists, master's-level counselors, therapists.

Q. Is there a place for the technicians?

A. Yes there is, with experience. And I can tell you, I started as a technician. I've done a variety of things. After graduating from college I started in a community mental health center; I worked as a case manager working with the chronics, monitoring their daily living, their medication, etc. And then I was a counselor at a partial or day hospital. Then I started moving to different areas. I worked at an inpatient (facility) as a psychiatric technician.

And at almost any hospital there are entry-level openings for individuals who've just finished a bachelor's degree or are in the process of finishing a bachelor's degree in psychology or social work, then get into those, working as a tech. However, as we've been saying, the field has been shifting, but still there will be a need, and it could be in an outpatient setting or in the chemical dependency field, too.

Q. What kind of people does your company need? Do you use technicians or only people with a B.A. and above?

A. B.A. and above. Many were technicians at one point. They realized they needed to do something else if they wanted to continue in the field. They needed to improve their degrees. The majority started as technicians, working in the education field as special education teachers and decided to go into a different part of the mental health area, occupational social work or EAP (employee assistance professional).

Q. Could you describe the concept of Employee Assistance Plans?

A. Employee assistance started as helping employers deal with troubled employees. And one of the things—it started way back, in the old days—was it was mainly someone who knew about alcoholism and substance abuse and they would assess the individual and get him into treatment and prevent the person from deteriorating more or have them to be fired. Now the employee assistance has shifted to a whole variety of services. From mental health crisis intervention, marital assistance, financial assistance, legal assistance. And we do serve our contracts with all varieties of services. The way it ties in with managed care is that in employee assistance we are into wellness. As employee assistance we provide quit smoking clinics, stress services, how to deal with troubled employees, how to recognize symptoms of depression or anxiety, things like that, just to give you a general idea. But the focus is to prevent. We are trying to avoid an illness, avoid spending a huge amount of dollars.

Q. How did you decide what education to get after you became a technician?

A. A lot of that was on-the-job training. I started again as a case manager with a bachelor's degree in psychology and social work, and since then I've been in a variety of mental health-related fields. The way I got into managed care was, I was working in an inpatient hospital in the late eighties, and I realized the shift was under way, and even though I was seeing a lot of patients staying for a long time, at the same time a lot of insurance companies were calling in and saying wait a minute, we need to do something about this. So I realized it was shifting and I needed to do something else.

And I started searching, and I knew there was another alternative to being in a hospital working the hours that I was working. And I began to do some research. I interviewed for a couple of positions in a managed care environment, and, of course, I checked into the one that was most beneficial to me and my family, and that was a large corporation, an insurance company that had a managed care component, and that's how I got into managed care. And in the last two years I have been in the EAP system.

Q. What is the fastest-growing sector of mental health care? Is it managed care and EAP?

A. I would say so, yes. Because it's combining in a way that it's not just to treat or to case manage the client. It's actually got a component of prevention. It's like the HMOs (health maintenance organization), which have a lot of preventive services. If we prevent the illness or at least teach people how to look at the signs, then we help people realize what alternatives they have before they get into trouble.

FOR MORE INFORMATION

Contact your state directors of mental health for information on public agencies and programs, private psychiatric hospitals in your area, and the National Association of Psychiatric Health Systems (202–393–6700) for a list of facilities in your area and special programs offered, such as alcohol treatment centers.

JOB PROFILES

HUMAN SERVICES WORKER

Other titles: Social service technician, case management aide, social work assistant, residential counselor, alcohol or drug abuse counselor, mental health technician, child abuse worker, community outreach worker, gerontology aide.

Work: Help clients obtain benefits or services; teach clients how to obtain services; monitor and keep case records.

Supervisor: Social worker, psychologist.

Workplace: Office, group residential facility.

Hours: Forty-hour week; some evenings or weekends. Shifts when in round-the-clock, twenty-four-hour care facilities.

Employment: 189,000 jobs 1992.

Training: High school adequate in some cases; most prefer college work in human services, social work, or social, behavioral science. 375 certificate, associate-degree programs available; 390 programs for bachelor's degree in human services. Master's degrees in human services administration.

Job outlook: Excellent. Field will grow through 2005.

Earnings: Starting salaries $12,000 to $20,000 in 1992. Experienced workers earn $15,000 to $25,000.

Related occupations: Social workers, community outreach workers, religious workers, occupational therapy assistants, physical therapy assistants, aides, psychiatric aides, activity leaders.

For More Information

Mary Di Giovanni RN, MS,
    Coordinator
    Council for Standards in Human
        Service Education
    Mental Health Technology
        Programs
    Northern Essex Community
        College
    Elliott Way
    Haverill, MA 01830

Douglas A. Whyte
    Community College of
        Philadelphia
    1700 Spring Garden Street
    Philadelphia, PA 19130-3991

Fitchburg State College
    Box #6257
    160 Pearl Street
    Fitchburg, MA 01420-2697

National Organization for Human
    Service Education
    Brookdale Community College
    Lyncroft, NJ 07738

See also regional affiliates.
    Note: Partial list of regional
        contacts available at community/
        state colleges.
    Source: *Occupational   Outlook
    Handbook,* 1994–95.

PSYCHIATRIC AIDES/MENTAL HEALTH WORKER

Other titles: Mental health assistants, psychiatric nursing assistants, ward attendants.

Work: Care for patients with mental illness or disability. Help with daily living activities: baths, dressing, grooming, meals. Lead them in social activities. Observe their behavior and report to professional staff as needed. Control unruly patients. Accompany patients to physicians for treatment.

Supervisor: Team may consist of psychiatrists, psychologists, psychiatric nurses, social workers, or therapists.

Workplace: Hospitals, state and county mental facilities, psychiatric units of general hospitals, private psychiatric facilities and community mental health centers, various outpatient settings, residential treatment centers.

Hours: Forty-hour week is usual. Because patients require care twenty-four hours a day, shift work is common.

Employment: 81,000 jobs in 1992.

Training: On-the-job training. Many employers do not require specific levels of education or experience. However, hospitals are often able to attract students in psychology programs. Associate degree programs in mental health technology are available from community colleges.

Job outlook: Better than average. Employment opportunities should rise with the aging of U.S. population. Many seniors require mental health services. Advancement depends on continuing education in psychology, social work, human services, special education, etc.

Earnings: Median salaries $13,800 in 1992. Top 10 percent earn more than $23,900.

For More information

Contact hospitals, nursing homes, psychiatric facilities, state boards of mental health, and state boards of nursing; and the National Association of State Mental Health Directors (703–739–9333). Also, see list of state mental health department human resources directors in Appendix B.

Source: *Occupation Outlook Handbook,* 1994–95.

RECREATIONAL THERAPIST, ACTIVITY DIRECTOR

Work: Plan activities that will improve the physical, mental, and emotional health of patients. Activities may be sports, art, music, dance, drama. Patients learn to socialize and build confidence. Therapists also keep records, lift and carry equipment, work with patients in recreation rooms or playing fields or swimming pools.

Supervisor: Hospital administrator, residential facilities, community mental health centers; some are self-employed, under contract to nursing homes or community agencies.

Workplace: About half of therapists work in hospitals. One-third work in nursing homes. Other health facilities and agencies also employ therapists.

Hours: Forty-hour week, plus some evenings and weekends.

Employment: 30,000 jobs in 1992.

Training: Associate degree in recreational therapy; bachelor's degree in therapeutic recreation is required for hospitals and clinical positions, usually. Training in art, drama, or music therapy is needed for therapy assistants; work experience may be acceptable substitute for degree for activity directors in some nursing homes.

Job outlook: Better than average. Growth is foreseen in long-term care, physical and psychiatric rehabilitation, and services for the disabled.

Earnings: Average salary was $25,500 in 1991. Average salary of activity directors is estimated between $15,000 and $25,000. Federal government therapist jobs paid an average $33,500 in 1993.

For More Information

American Therapeutic Recreation
    Association
    c/o Associated Management
      Systems
P.O. Box 15215
Hattiesburg, MS 39402-5215

National Council for Therapeutic
    Recreation Certification

P.O. Box 479
Thiells, NY 10984-0479

National Therapeutic Recreation
    Society
2775 South Quincy Street, Ste. 300
Arlington, VA 22206-2204

Source: *Occupational Outlook Handbook,* 1994–95.

LICENSED PRACTICAL NURSE, LICENSED VOCATIONAL NURSE

Work: LPNs with psychiatric training work in hospitals, nursing homes, and home health settings. They care for patients and where they're licensed to, they provide medication to patients.

Supervisor: RN or a more experienced LPN; physician in clinic or hospital setting.

Workplace: Hospital, nursing home, clinic, patients' homes.

Hours: Forty-hour week, sometimes as part of three shift schedule in hospital and twenty-four-hour care facilities. Private duty nurses can set their own work hours.

Employment: All LPNs held 659,000 jobs in 1992. Most were in medical surgical positions. Perhaps 10 percent would have had a mental health component to their jobs.

Training: LPNs must pass state-mandated licensing exams. To prepare for the exams, most students enroll in a one-year preparatory program. A high school diploma is required to enter this program. Practical nursing training programs include classroom work and supervised clinical practice. In addition to basic nursing, students learn anatomy, physiology, medical-surgical nursing, pediatrics, and psychiatric nursing, among other studies.

Job outlook: Excellent, according to government forecasts. Job prospects are best in nursing homes; rapid growth is expected in residential care facilities, including group homes for the mentally retarded. Hospital employment will remain stable.

Earnings: Median earnings of full-time LPNs were $21,476 in 1992. Top 10 percent earned more than $31,668.

For More Information

American Nurses' Association
  600 Maryland Avenue SW
  Washington, DC 20024-2571

American Psychiatric Nurses
    Association
  1200 Nineteenth Street NW
  Suite 300
  Washington, DC 20036

  (Professional society for practicing nurses)

National Association for Practical
    Nurse Education and Service,
    Inc.
  1400 Spring Street, Suite 310
  Silver Spring, MD 20910

  For information on LPN programs.

National Association of State Mental
    Health Directors
  66 Canal Center Plaza
  Suite 302
  Alexandria, VA 22314

National Federation of Licensed
    Practical Nurses, Inc.
  P.O. Box 18088
  Raleigh, NC 27619

  Contact also state departments of mental health for information on licensing.

  Source: *Occupational Outlook Handbook,* 1994–95.

HOMEMAKER-HOME HEALTH AIDE

Work: Give personal care to patients at home. Provide psychological support. Observe patient. Monitor living conditions. Assist with treatment as prescribed by nurse, physician, and mental health team. Offer psychological support to patient.

Supervisor: Nurse coordinator, registered nurse, physical therapist, or social worker.

Workplace: Patients' homes, agency office. Employed by home health agencies, visiting nurse associations, public health and welfare departments, community volunteer agencies.

Hours: Variable. Usually an eight-hour day, four or five clients per day. Same clients may be seen for years.

Employment: 475,000 jobs in 1992.

Training: Federal guidelines for Medicare patients with mental health diagnoses. At least seventy-five hours of classroom and practical training. Certification is available. State certification requirements apply. Some community colleges offer psychiatric component to training of home health aides. Some agencies require (CNA) certified nurses aide or B.S.N. nursing degree, especially where medication is required.

Job outlook: One of the fastest growing occupations through 2005, more than doubling due to rapid growth and high turnover in the field.

Earnings: Hourly wage was $6.31 for starting workers, $8.28 for experienced workers in 1992.

Related occupations: Child monitors, occupational therapy aides, psychiatric aides.

For More Information

Foundation for Hospice and Homecare/National Certification Program
519 C Street NE
Washington, DC 20002
Includes the former National HomeCaring Council.
Source: *Occupational Outlook Handbook,* 1994–95.

SOCIAL WORKER

Work: Mental health social workers help clients through group therapy, one-to-one therapy sessions, crisis intervention, social rehabilitation, and skills in activities of daily living.

Supervisor: Psychologist, psychiatrist, or other member of mental health team.

Workplace: Community center; state, county, or municipal government agency; in office or in local travel for community outreach and client visits.

Hours: Forty-hour week, some evenings and weekends for client appointments, community meetings, crises.

Employment: 484,000 jobs in 1992. Forty percent with governmental agencies; others in private sector with social services, community or religious organizations, hospitals, nursing homes, home health agencies.

Training: Bachelor's degree required for most jobs. Master's degree in social work is preferred, especially for mental health settings. B.S.W. programs include 400 hours of supervised field experience. M.S.W. takes two years and 900 hours of fieldwork.

Job outlook: Better than average through 2005. More social services for seniors will be needed. Services are needed for the mentally ill, retarded, and those in crisis.

Earnings: B.S.W. earnings $20,000 a year; M.S.W. $30,000 in 1992.

For More Information

National Association of Social Workers
    750 First Street NE
    Suite 700
    Washington, DC 20002-4241

A directory of accredited B.S.W. and S.W. programs is available for $10 from:

Council on Social Work Education
    1600 Duke Street
    Alexandria, VA 22314-3421

COUNSELOR

Work: Mental health counselors work to promote good mental health in the community, with an emphasis on prevention of problems. They deal with substance abuse, domestic and marital problems, stress management, suicide, aging, job and career concerns, education decisions, and other issues.

Supervisor: Supervisor or administrator of a mental health agency; some counselors are self-employed or work with and for psychologists, psychiatrists, clinical social workers.

Workplace: Mental health agency, community agencies.

Hours: Forty-hour week with evening appointments for clients.

Employment: Overall employment is likely to grow faster than average through 2005. Rehabilitation and mental health counselors will be in strong demand.

Training: Mental health counselors need a master's degree in mental health counseling, psychology, or social work. Certification is available through the National Board of Certified Clinical Mental Health Counselors. Continuing education to maintain certification.

Job outlook: Faster than average growth is expected through 2005.

Earnings: $30,000 median earnings for school and vocational counselors.

For More Information

American Counseling Association
5999 Stevenson Avenue
Alexandria, VA 22304

For a list of accredited educational programs, contact ACA's Council for Accreditation of Counseling and Related Educational Programs.

American Mental Health Counselors Association, American Counseling Association
5999 Stevenson Avenue
Alexandria, VA 22304

For information on mental health counseling.

National Association of Alcoholism and Drug Abuse Counselors
3717 Columbia Pike, Suite 300
Arlington, VA 22204

For information about drug abuse and alcohol counseling.

National Council on Alcoholism and Drug Dependence Inc.
12 West Twenty-First Street
New York, NY 10010

NURSE'S AIDE, NURSING ATTENDANT, CERTIFIED NURSE'S AIDE

Work: Help older patients who are physically and/or mentally ill.

Supervisor: Nurse, director of nursing.

Workplace: Nursing home, congregate care home, assisted living facility.

Hours: Standard three-shift rotation. Flexible night and weekend hours can help those who want to work while they attend school.

Employment: 650,000 in nursing homes, others in halfway houses or in private households (see also home health aide).

Training: In some cases, no training required prior to starting. On-the-job training at a nursing home will include mandatory training and a competency test within four months to be placed on the state registry of nursing aides. Additional training is offered in high schools, vocational-technical schools, community colleges. Personal care skills for disabled patients include bathing, feeding, and grooming. Aides also need to know about nutrition, anatomy, infection control, and other subjects.

Job outlook: Very good through 2005. Much faster than average growth due to fast-growing population of senior citizens in need of nursing care.

Earnings: Median annual earnings $13,800 in 1992. Nursing aides in chain nursing homes, $11,600 median annual according to Buck Survey in January 1993.

For More Information

American Association of Homes for
the Aging
901 E Street NW, Suite 500
Washington, DC 20004-2037

American Nurses' Association
600 Maryland Avenue SW,
Suite 100 W
Washington, DC 20024-2571

Foundation for Hospice and
Homecare/National Certification
Program
519 C Street NE
Washington, DC 20002
Includes the former National Home-
Caring Council.

STATE MENTAL HEALTH DESIGNATED REPRESENTATIVES FOR HUMAN RESOURCES*

Alabama

Director of Human Resources
    Management
Department of Mental Health &
    Mental Retardation
200 Interstate Park Dr., P.O. 3710
Montgomery, AL 36193-50001

Alaska

Project Director for Human Resource
    Development
Division of Mental Health &
    Developmental Disabilities
Department of Health & Social
    Services
Pouch H-04
Juneau, AK 99811

American Samoa

Chief, Social Services Division
    Department of Human Resources
American Samoa Government
Pago Pago, American Samoa
    96799

Arizona

Manager, Office of Planning, Rules &
    Grants
ADHS/Behavioral Health Services
2122 E. Highland, Ste. 100
Phoenix, AZ 85016

Arkansas

Director for Human Resources
    Department of Human Services
Division of Mental Health Services
4313 West Markham Street
Little Rock, AR 72205-4096

California

Deputy Director
    Systems of Care Division
Department of Mental Health
1600 9th Street, Room 250
Sacramento, CA 95814

Colorado

Director
    Planning & Staff Development
Division of Mental Health

---

*Source: National Association of State Mental Health Program Directors, October 1994 list.

Department of Institutions
3520 West Oxford Avenue
Denver, CO 80236

Connecticut

Director of Human Resource
    Development
    90 Washington Street
    Hartford, CT 06106

Delaware

Director, Div. of Community Planning
    & Program Development &
    Training
    Division of Alcohol, Drug Abuse
    & Mental Health
    Department of Health & Social
    Services
    1901 North DuPont Highway
    New Castle, DE 19720

District of Columbia

Chief, Planning & Evaluation
    Division
    Department of Human Services
    Commission on Mental Health
    Services
    Behavioral Studies Building, #222,
    S.E.
    2700 Martin Luther King, Jr.
    Avenue
    Washington, DC 20032

Florida

Human Services Program Specialist
    Alcohol, Drug Abuse & Mental
    Health Program Office
    1317 Winewood Boulevard
    Tallahassee, FL 32301

Georgia

Director, Resource Management &
    Development Section

Division of Mental Health, Mental
    Retardation & Substance Abuse
    878 Peachtree Street, N.E. #309
    Atlanta, GA 30309

Guam

Director
    Department of Mental Health &
    Substance Abuse
    P.O. Box 9400
    Tanuning, Guam 96911

Hawaii

Assistant Chief
    Adult Mental Health Division
    Department of Health
    1250 Punchbowl Street, Suite 256
    P.O. Box 3378
    Honolulu, HI 96801

Idaho

Assistant Administrator
    Division of Community
        Rehabilitation
    Department of Health & Welfare
    450 West State Street
    Statehouse Mail
    Boise, ID 83720

Illinois

Director of HRD
    Department of Mental Health &
        Developmental Disabilities
    State of Illinois Building
    160 North La Salle, Ste. 1000
    Chicago, IL 60601

Indiana

Director
    Human Resource Administration
    Family & Social Services
    Division of Mental Health
    302 West Washington Street, E-431
    Indianapolis, IN 46204-2739

Iowa

HRD Specialist
  Division of Mental Health, Mental
    Retardation & Developmental
    Disabilities
  Department of Human Services
  Hoover State Office Building
  East 12th & Walnut Streets
  Des Moines, IA 50319

Kansas

Education Program Specialist
  Mental Health & Retardation
    Services
  Department of Social &
    Rehabilitation Services
  Docking State Office Building
  5th Floor North
  10th and Topeka Streets
  Topeka, KS 66612

Kentucky

Director
  Human Resource Development
  Department for Mental Health &
    Mental Retardation Services
  275 East Main Street
  Frankfort, KY 40621

Louisiana

Department of Health & Hospitals
  Office of Human Services
  P.O. Box 3018
  Baton Rouge, LA 70821

Maine

Human Resource Division
  Department of Mental Health &
    Mental Retardation
  411 State Office Building
  Station 40
  Augusta, ME 04333

Maryland

Chief, Division of Human Resource
    Development
  Mental Hygiene Administration
  Department of Health & Mental
    Hygiene
  201 West Preston Street
  State Office Building
  Baltimore, MD 21201

Massachusetts

Director of Staff Training &
    Development
  Department of Mental Health
  25 Staniford Street, Central Office
  Boston, MA 02114

Michigan

Director for Administration
  Department of Mental Health
  Lewis-Cass Building
  320 Walnut Boulevard
  Lansing, MI 48913

Minnesota

Director of Human Resource
    Development Project
  Department of Human Services
  Mental Health Division
  444 Lafayette Road
  St. Paul, MN 55155-3828

Mississippi

Director of Human Resource Division
  Department of Mental Health
  1101 Robert E. Lee Building
  239 North Lamar Street
  Jackson, MS 39201

Missouri

Deputy Director for Human
    Resources
Department of Mental Health
1706 East Elm Street
P.O. Box 687
Jefferson City, MO 65102

Montana

Human Resource Development
    Project Director
Mental Health Division
Department of Corrections and
    Human Services
1539 Eleventh Avenue
Helena, MT 59620

Nebraska

Resource Development & Training
    Director
Department of Public Institutions
P.O. Box 8-94728
Lincoln, NE 68509

Nevada

Division of Mental Hygiene & Mental
    Retardation
Department of Human Resources
Gilbert Building, Ste. 1-H
1001 North Mountain Street
Carson City, NV 89710

New Hampshire

Coordinator
    Office of Human Resource
        Development
    Division of Mental Health &
        Developmental Services
    State Office Park S., 105 Pleasant
        Street
    Concord, NH 03301

New Jersey

Office of Human Resources
    Division of Mental Health &
        Hospitals
    Department of Human Services
    50 E. State Street, Capitol Center,
        CN 727
    Trenton, NJ 08625-0727

New Mexico

Director of Human Resources
    Health & Environment Department
    1190 St. Francis Drive
    Room N-3211, P.O. Box 968
    Santa Fe, NM 87503

New York

Deputy Commissioner
    Clinical Support Division
    Office of Mental Health
    44 Holland Avenue
    Albany, NY 12229

North Carolina

Coordinator, Mental Health Services
    for the Elderly
    Division of Mental Health, Mental
        Retardation & Substance Abuse
        Services
    Department of Human Resources
    325 North Salisbury Street
    Raleigh, NC 27611

North Dakota

Director
    Division of Mental Health
    Office of Human Services
    Department of Human Services
    State Capitol Building
    Bismarck, ND 58505

Ohio

Chief
  Office of Education & Training
  Department of Mental Health
  30 East Broad Street
  Columbus, OH 43215

Oklahoma

Coordinator of Human Resource
    Development
  Department of Mental Health
  P.O. Box 53277, Capitol Station
  Oklahoma City, OK 73152

Oregon

Office of Mental Health Services
  Mental Health & Developmental
    Disability Services Division
  Department of Human Resources
  2575 Bittern Street, N.E.
  Salem, OR 97310

Pennsylvania

Chief, Division of Planning & Human
    Resource Development
  Department of Public Health
  Office of Mental Health
  P.O. Box 2675
  Harrisburg, PA 17105-2675

Puerto Rico

Assistant Secretary for Mental Health
  Department of Health
  G.P.O. Box 61
  San Juan, Puerto Rico 00936

Rhode Island

Assistant Director for Human
    Resource Development
  Department of Mental Health,
    Mental Retardation & Hospitals
  600 New London Avenue
  Cranston, RI 02920

South Carolina

Coordinator for Human Resource
    Development
  Department of Mental Health
  2414 Bull Street, P.O. Box 485
  Columbia, SC 29202

South Dakota

Director
  Office of Mental Health &
    Developmental Disabilities
  Department of Social Services
  East Highway 34, 500 East Capitol
  Pierre, SD 57501

Tennessee

Director for Human Resource
    Development
  Division of Mental Health &
    Mental Retardation
  11th Floor, Gateway Towers
  710 James Robertson Parkway
  Nashville, Tennessee 37243

Texas

Director, Human Resources Services
  Department of Mental Health &
    Mental Retardation
  P.O. Box 12668, Capitol Station
  Austin, TX 78711

Utah

Assistant Director
  Division of Mental Health
  Department of Social Services
  120 North, 200 West, 4th Floor
  Salt Lake City, UT 84103

Vermont

Director of Planning
  Department of Mental Health
  103 South Main Street
  Waterbury, VT 05676

Virginia

Director for Human Resource
    Development
    Division of Mental Health Services
    Department of Mental Health &
    Mental Retardation
    109 Governor Street
    Richmond, VA 23214

Virgin Islands

Assistant Director, Research, Planning
    and Special Programs
    Division of Mental Health,
    Alcoholism & Drug
    Dependency, Department of
    Health
    P.O. Box 520
    St. Croix, U.S. Virgin Islands
    00820

Washington

Clinical Professor, The Washington
    Institute for MI Research &
    Training
    University of Washington
    P.O. Box 94500, Western Branch
    Ft. Stellacoom, WA 98494-0500

West Virginia

Office of Behavioral Health Services
    Division of Health
    Building 3, Room 451
    1900 Kanawha Boulevard East
    Charleston, WV 25305

Wisconsin

Director of Human Resource
    Development
    Office of Mental Health
    P.O. Box 7851, 1 W. Wilson Street,
    Rm. 443
    Madison, WI 53707-7851

Wyoming

Mental Health Program Manager
    Division of Behavioral Health
    Department of Health
    450 Hathaway Building
    Cheyenne, WY 82002